THE

M000205534

James H. O'Keefe, Jr., MD, FACC
Professor of Medicine
University of Missouri, Kansas City
Director, Preventive Cardiology
Mid-America Heart Institute
St. Luke's Hospital
Kansas City, Missouri

Stephen C. Hammill, MD, FACC, FHRS
Past President, Heart Rhythm Society
Professor of Medicine
Director, Electrocardiography Laboratories
Mayo Clinic
Rochester, Minnesota

Mark S. Freed, MD, FACC
Cardiologist
Chicago, Illinois
Founder and Past President
Physicians' Press

Steven M. Pogwizd, MD, FACC
Featheringill Endowed Professor in Cardiac Arrhythmia Research
Professor of Medicine, Physiology & Biophysics, and Biomedical Engineering
Associate Director, Cardiac Rhythm Management Laboratory
The University of Alabama at Birmingham
Birmingham, Alabama

PHYSICIANS' PRESS
AN IMPRINT OF JONES AND BARTLETT PUBLISHERS
Sudbury, Massachusetts
BOSTON   TORONTO   LONDON   SINGAPORE

World Headquarters

Jones and Bartlett Publishers	Jones and Bartlett Publishers	Jones and Bartlett Publishers
40 Tall Pine Drive	Canada	International
Sudbury, MA 01776	6339 Ormindale Way	Barb House, Barb Mews
978-443-5000	Mississauga, Ontario L5V 1J2	London W6 7PA
info@jbpub.com	Canada	United Kingdom
www.jbpub.com		

Jones and Bartlett's books and products are available through most bookstores and online booksellers. To contact Jones and Bartlett Publishers directly, call 800-832-0034, fax 978-443-8000, or visit our website, www.jbpub.com.

Substantial discounts on bulk quantities of Jones and Bartlett's publications are available to corporations, professional associations, and other qualified organizations. For details and specific discount information, contact the special sales department at Jones and Bartlett via the above contact information or send an email to specialsales@jbpub.com.

Production Credits

Senior Acquisitions Editor: Alison Hankey
Editorial Assistant: Sara Cameron
Production Assistant: Lisa Lamenzo
Senior Marketing Manager: Barb Bartoszek
V.P., Manufacturing and Inventory Control: Therese Connell
Composition: Publishers' Design and Production Services, Inc.
Cover Design: Scott Moden
Cover Image: © Jones and Bartlett Publishers, LLC
Printing and Binding: Cenveo
Cover Printing: Cenveo

Library of Congress Cataloging-in-Publication Data
The ECG criteria book / James H. O'Keefe Jr. ... [et al.]. — 2nd ed.
  p. ; cm.
Includes index.
ISBN 978-0-7637-6252-0
1. Electrocardiography. 2. Heart—Diseases—Diagnosis. I. O'Keefe, James H.
[DNLM: 1. Electrocardiography. 2. Heart Diseases—diagnosis. WG 140 E1678 2010]
RC683.5.E5E243 2010
616.1'207547—dc22

2009032463

6048

TABLE OF CONTENTS

ABBREVIATIONS

APC	Atrial premature complex
AV	Atrioventricular
bpm	Beats per minute
COPD	Chronic obstructive pulmonary disease
ECG	Electrocardiogram
IVCD	Intraventricular conduction disturbance
JPC	Junctional premature complex
LAFB	Left anterior fascicular block
LBBB	Left bundle branch block
LPFB	Left posterior fascicular block
LVH	Left ventricular hypertrophy
MI	Myocardial infarction
RBBB	Right bundle branch block
RVH	Right ventricular hypertrophy
SA	Sinoatrial
SVT	Supraventricular tachycardia
VA	Ventriculoatrial
VF	Ventricular fibrillation
VPC	Ventricular premature complex
VT	Ventricular tachycardia
WPW	Wolff-Parkinson-White

Nomenclature

The relative amplitudes of the component waves of the QRS complex are described using small (lowercase) and large (uppercase) letters. For example, an *rS complex* describes a QRS with a small R wave and a large S wave; a *qRs complex* describes a QRS with a small Q wave, a large R wave, and a small S wave; and an *RSR′ complex* describes a QRS with a large R wave, a large S wave, and a large secondary R wave (R′). When the QRS complex consists solely of a Q wave, a *QS* designation is used.

— Section 1 —

APPROACH TO
ECG INTERPRETATION

Each ECG should be read in a thorough and systematic fashion. It is important to be organized, compulsive, and strict in your application of the ECG criteria. Analyze the following features on every ECG:

Section 1 Approach to ECG Interpretation

Once these features have been identified, ask the following questions:

1. Is an arrhythmia or conduction disturbance present?
2. Is chamber enlargement or hypertrophy present?
3. Is ischemia, injury, or infarction present?
4. Is a clinical disorder present?

Be sure to consider each ECG in the context of the clinical history. For example, diffuse mild ST-segment elevation in a young, asymptomatic patient without previous cardiac history is likely to represent early repolarization abnormality, whereas the same finding in a patient with chest pain and a friction rub is more likely to represent acute pericarditis.

1. Heart Rate

The following method can be used to determine heart rate (assumes a standard paper speed of 25 mm/sec).

Regular Rhythm

- Count the number of large boxes between P waves (atrial rate), R waves (ventricular rate), or pacer spikes (pacemaker rate).
- Beats per minute = 300 divided by the number of large boxes.

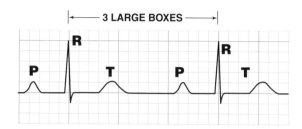

Heart Rate = 300 ⨸ no. large boxes between "R" Waves = 300 ⨸ 3 = 100 bpm

Note: It is easier to memorize the heart rates associated with each of the large boxes, rather than counting the number of large boxes (1, 2, 3, etc.) and dividing into 300:

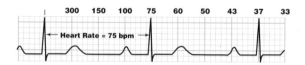

Section 1 Approach to ECG Interpretation

Note: If the number of large boxes is not a whole number, either estimate the rate (this is routine practice) or divide 1500 by the number of small boxes between P waves (atrial rate), R waves (ventricular rate), or pacer spikes (pacemaker rate):

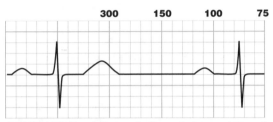

ESTIMATED Heart Rate = halfway between 100 and 75 = ~ 87 bpm (or 1500 ÷ 17.5 small boxes)

Note: For tachycardias, it is helpful to memorize the rates between 150 and 300 bpm:

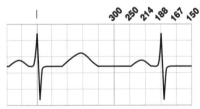

Heart Rate = 188 bpm

Slow or Irregular Rhythm

- Identify the 3-second markers at top or bottom of ECG tracing.
- Count the number of QRS complexes (or P waves or pacer spikes) that appear in 6 seconds (i.e., two consecutive 3-second markers).
- Multiply by 10 to obtain rate in bpm.

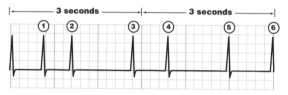

ESTIMATED Heart Rate = number of QRS complexes in 6 seconds x 10 = 6 x 10 = 60 bpm

2. P Wave

What It Represents

The P wave represents electrical forces generated from atrial activation. The first and second halves of the P wave roughly correspond to right and left atrial activation, respectively.

What to Measure

- Duration (seconds): Measured from the beginning of P wave to the end of P wave.

- Amplitude (mm): Measured from baseline to top (or bottom) of P wave. Positive and negative deflections are determined separately. One small box = 1 mm on standard scale ECGs (i.e., 10 mm = 1 mV).

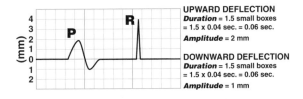

- Morphology:

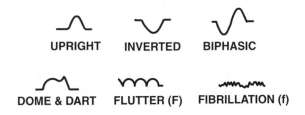

P-Wave Characteristics

- Normal P-wave duration: 0.08–0.11 second
- Normal P-wave axis: 0–75°
- Normal P-wave morphology: Upright in I, II, aVF; upright or biphasic in III, aVL, V_1, V_2; small notching may be present
- Normal P-wave amplitude: Limb leads: < 2.5 mm; V_1: positive deflection < 1.5 mm and negative deflection < 1 mm

3. Origin of the Rhythm

Rhythm identification is one of the most difficult and complex aspects of ECG interpretation, and it is also one of the most common mistakes made by computer ECG interpretation programs. Proper rhythm interpretation requires integration of heart rate, R-R regularity, P-wave morphology, PR interval, QRS width, and the P:QRS relationship. No single algorithm can simply describe all the various permutations; however, the following rhythm-recognition tables, based initially on the P:QRS relationship and heart rate, provide a useful frame of reference:

P:QRS Relationships

P:QRS < 1: Junctional or ventricular premature complexes or rhythms (escape, accelerated, tachycardia)

P:QRS = 1

- *P wave precedes QRS:* Sinus rhythm; ectopic atrial rhythm; multifocal atrial tachycardia; wandering atrial pacemaker; SVT (sinus node reentry tachycardia, automatic atrial tachycardia); sinoatrial exit block, 2°; conducted APCs with any of the above

- *P wave follows QRS:* SVT (AV nodal reentry tachycardia, orthodromic SVT); junctional or ventricular rhythm with 1:1 retrograde atrial activation

  No P Waves: Atrial fibrillation; atrial flutter; sinus arrest with junctional or ventricular escape rhythm;

SVT (AV nodal reentry tachycardia, AV reentry tachy-cardia), junctional tachycardia or VT with P wave buried in QRS; VF

Heart Rate < 100 bpm

Narrow QRS (< 0.12 second)—Regular R-R

- Sinus P; rate 60–100: *Sinus rhythm*
- Sinus P; rate < 60: *Sinus bradycardia*
- Nonsinus P; PR ≥ 0.12: *Ectopic atrial rhythm*
- Nonsinus P; PR < 0.12: *Junctional or low atrial rhythm*
- Sawtooth flutter waves: *Atrial flutter, usually with 4:1 AV block*
- No P; rate < 60: *Junctional rhythm*
- No P; rate 60–100: *Accelerated junctional rhythm*

Narrow QRS—Irregular R-R

- Sinus P; P-P varying > 0.16 second: *Sinus arrhythmia*
- Sinus and nonsinus P: *Wandering atrial pacemaker*
- *Any regular rhythm with 2° or 3° AV block or premature beats*
- Fine or coarse baseline oscillations: *Atrial fibrillation with slow ventricular response*
- Sawtooth flutter waves: *Atrial flutter, usually with variable AV block*
- P:QRS ratio > 1: *2° or 3° AV block or blocked APCs*

- P:QRS ratio < 1: *Junctional or ventricular premature beats or escape rhythm*

Wide QRS (≥ 0.12 second)

- Sinus or nonsinus P: *Any supraventricular rhythm with a preexisting IVCD (e.g., bundle branch block) or aberrancy*
- No P†; rate < 60: *Idioventricular rhythm*
- No P†; rate 60–100: *Accelerated idioventricular rhythm*

† AV dissociation may be present

Heart Rate > 100 bpm

Narrow QRS (< 0.12 second)—Regular R-R

- Sinus P: *Sinus tachycardia*
- Flutter waves: *Atrial flutter*
- No P: *AV nodal reentrant tachycardia (AVNRT), junctional tachycardia*
- Short R-P (R-P < 50% of R-R interval): *AVNRT, orthodromic SVT (AVRT), atrial tachycardia with 1° AV block, junctional tachycardia with 1:1 retrograde atrial activation*
- Long R-P (R-P > 50% of R-R interval): *Atrial tachycardia, sinus node reentrant tachycardia, atypical AVNRT, orthodromic SVT with prolonged V-A conduction*

Narrow QRS—Irregular R-R

- Nonsinus P; > 3 morphologies: *Multifocal atrial tachycardia*
- Fine or coarse baseline oscillations: *Atrial fibrillation*
- Flutter waves: *Atrial flutter*
- *Any regular rhythm with 2° or 3° AV block or premature beats*

Wide QRS (≥ 0.12 second)

- Sinus or nonsinus P: *Any regular or irregular supraventricular rhythm with a preexisting IVCD or aberrancy*
- No P; rate 100–110: *Accelerated idioventricular rhythm*
- No P; rate 110–250: *VT, SVT with aberrancy*
- Irregular, polymorphic, alternating polarity: *Torsade de pointes*
- Chaotic irregular oscillations; no discrete QRS: *Ventricular fibrillation*

4. PR Interval and Segment

What It Represents

- PR interval represents conduction time from the onset of atrial depolarization to the onset of ventricular repolarization. It does not reflect conduction from the sinus node to the atrium.

- PR segment represents atrial repolarization.

How to Measure

- PR interval (seconds): From the beginning of the P wave to the first deflection of the QRS complex. Measure longest PR seen.

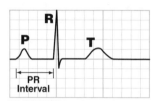

PR INTERVAL = 4 small boxes =
4 x 0.04 = 0.16 sec.

- PR segment (mm): Amount of elevation or depression relative to the TP segment (end of the T wave to the beginning of the P wave).

Definitions
PR Interval

- Normal PR interval: 0.12–0.20 second
- Prolonged PR interval: > 0.20 second
- Short PR interval: < 0.12 second

PR Segment

- Normal PR segment: Usually isoelectric. May be displaced in a direction opposite to the P wave. Elevation is usually < 0.5 mm; depression is usually < 0.8 mm.
- PR-segment elevation: Usually ≥ 0.5 mm
- PR-segment depression: Usually ≥ 0.8 mm

5. QRS Duration

What It Represents

Duration of ventricular activation

How to Measure

In seconds, from the beginning to the end of the QRS (or QS) complex

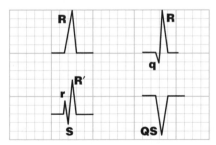

QRS duration = 1.5 small boxes = 0.06 sec.

Definitions

- Normal QRS duration: < 0.10 second
- Increased QRS duration: ≥ 0.10 second

  Note: For the purposes of establishing a differential diagnosis, it is often useful to distinguish moderate prolongation of the QRS (0.10 to ≤ 0.12 second) from marked prolongation of the QRS (> 0.12 second).

6. QT Interval

What It Represents

Total duration of ventricular systole—i.e., ventricular depolarization (QRS complex) and repolarization (T wave)

How to Measure

- QT interval: In seconds, from the beginning of the QRS (or QS) complex to the end of the T wave. It is best to use a lead with a large T wave and distinct termination (often leads II and V2).

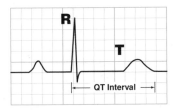

**QT interval = 8 small boxes =
8 x 0.04 sec. = 0.32 sec.**

- Corrected QT interval (QTc): Since the normal QT interval varies inversely with heart rate, the QTc, which corrects for heart rate, is usually determined.
  - ▸ QTc (seconds) = QT interval (seconds) divided by the square root of the preceding R-R interval (seconds). *Example*: For heart rate of 50 bpm, R-R interval = 1.2 seconds, and QTc = QT ÷ square root of 1.2 = QT ÷ 1.1.
  - ▸ Alternative method: Use 0.40 second as the normal QT interval for a heart rate of 70 bpm. For every 10 bpm change in heart rate above (or below) 70, subtract (or add) 0.02 second. The measured value should be within ± 0.04 second of the calculated normal. *Example*: For a heart rate of 100 bpm, the calculated "normal" QT interval = 0.40 second – (3 × 0.02 second) = 0.34 ± 0.04 second. For a heart rate of 50 bpm, the calculated "normal" QT interval = 0.40 second + (2 × 0.02 second) = 0.44 ± 0.04 second.

Definitions

- Normal QTc: 0.30–0.44 second for heart rates of 60–100 bpm. The normal QT should be < 50% of the R-R interval.
- Prolonged QTc: ≥ 0.45 second
- Short QTc: < 0.30 second for heart rates of 60–100 bpm

7. QRS Axis

What It Represents

The major vector of ventricular activation

How to Determine

- Determine if "net QRS voltage" (upward minus downward QRS deflection) is positive (> 0) or negative (< 0) in leads I, II, aVF:

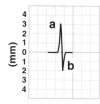

NET QRS VOLTAGE =
upward – downward deflection (mm)
= a – b = 3 – 2 = 1 (positive)

Section 1 Approach to ECG Interpretation

• Determine axis category according to the following chart:

Table 1			
Axis	**Net QRS voltage**		
	Lead I	**aVF**	**Lead II**
Normal axis (0° to +90°)	+	+	
Normal variant (0° to –30°)	+	–	+
Left axis deviation (–30° to –90°)	+	–	–
Right axis deviation (> 100°)	–	+	
Right superior axis (–90° to +180°)	–	–	
+ represents positive (> 0) net QRS voltage – represents negative (< 0) net QRS voltage			

8. QRS Voltage

How to Measure

In millimeters, from baseline to the peak of the R wave (R-wave voltage) or S wave (S-wave voltage) (see QRS axis in previous section)

Definitions

- Normal voltage: Amplitude of the QRS has a wide range of normal limits, depending on the lead, age of the individual, and other factors.

- Low voltage (from peak of R wave to peak of S wave): Total QRS amplitude (R + S) < 5 mm in all limb leads and < 10 mm in all precordial leads.

- Increased voltage: See LVH (item 40, Section 3) and RVH (item 41, Section 3).

9. R-Wave Progression

How to Identify

Determine the *precordial transition zone*—i.e., the lead with equal R- and S-wave voltage (R/S = 1)

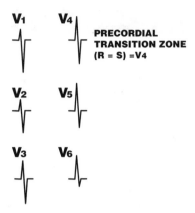

Definitions

- Normal R-wave progression: Transition zone = V_2–V_4, with increasing R-wave amplitude across the precordial leads. (Exception: R wave in V_5 often exceeds R wave in V_6.)
- Poor R-wave progression: Transition zone = V_5 or V_6
- Reverse R-wave progression: Decreasing R-wave amplitude across the precordial leads

10. Q Wave

How to Identify

A Q wave is present when the first deflection of the QRS is negative. If the QRS consists exclusively of a negative deflection, that deflection is considered a Q wave, but the complex is referred to as a "QS" complex.

What to Measure

Duration, in seconds, from the beginning to the end (i.e., when it returns to baseline) of the Q wave. When the QRS complex consists solely of a Q wave, a "QS" designation is used.

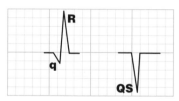

Q wave duration = 1 small box
= 0.04 seconds

Definitions

- Normal Q waves: Small Q waves (duration < 0.03 second) are common in most leads, except aVR, V_1–V_3.
- Abnormal Q waves: Any Q wave in leads V_1–V_3. Q wave ≥ 0.03 second in leads I, II, aVL, aVF, V_4, V_5, or V_6. **Note**: For Q-wave myocardial infarction, Q-wave changes must

be present in at least two contiguous leads and must be ≥ 1 mm in depth.

11. ST Segment

What It Represents

The ST segment represents the interval between the end of ventricular depolarization (QRS complex) and the beginning of depolarization (T wave). It is identified as the segment between the end of the QRS complex and the beginning of the T wave.

What to Identify

- Amount of elevation or depression, in millimeters, relative to the TP segment (end of the T wave to the beginning of the P wave)

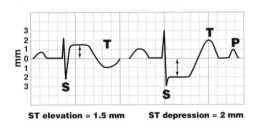

ST elevation = 1.5 mm   ST depression = 2 mm

- ST-segment morphology:

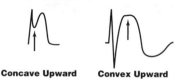

Concave Upward   **Convex Upward**

ST DEPRESSION:

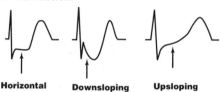

Horizontal   **Downsloping**   **Upsloping**

Definitions

- Normal ST segment: Usually isoelectric, but may vary from 0.5 mm below to 1 mm above baseline in limb leads, and up to 3 mm concave upward elevation may be seen in the precordial leads in early repolarization (see item 61, Section 3).

  Note: While some ST-segment depression and elevation can be seen in normals, it may also indicate myocardial infarction, injury, or some other pathological process. It is especially important to consider the clinical presentation and to compare it to previous ECGs (if available) when ST-segment depression or elevation is identified.

- Nonspecific ST segment: Slight (< 1 mm) ST-segment depression or elevation.

12. T Wave

What It Represents

The electrical forces generated from ventricular repolarization

What to Identify

- Amplitude: In millimeters, from baseline to peak or valley of the T wave:

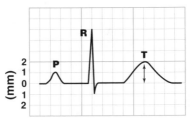

T wave amplitude = 2 mm

- Morphology:

UPRIGHT   PEAKED   INVERTED

NOTCHED   BIPHASIC

— 22 —

Definitions

- Normal T-wave morphology: Upright in I, II, V_3–V_6; inverted in aVR, V_1; may be upright, flat, or biphasic in III, aVL, aVF, V_1, V_2. T-wave inversion may be present in V_1–V_3 in healthy young adults (for juvenile T waves, see item 62, Section 3).

- Normal T-wave amplitude: Usually < 6 mm in limb leads and ≤ 10 mm in precordial leads

- Tall T waves: Amplitude > 6 mm in limb leads or > 10 mm in precordial leads

- Nonspecific T waves: Flat or slightly inverted

13. U Wave

What It Represents

Controversial: Afterpotentials of ventricular muscle vs. repolarization of Purkinje fibers

How to Identify

When present, the U wave manifests as a small (usually positive) deflection following the T wave. At faster heart rates, the U wave may be superimposed on the preceding T wave.

What to Determine

- Morphology: upright, inverted, or absent
- Height, in millimeters, from baseline to peak or valley

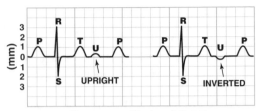

U wave amplitude = 0.3 mm

Definitions

- Normal U wave: Not always present. Morphology is upright in all leads except aVR. Amplitude is 5–25% the height of the T wave (usually < 1.5 mm). U waves are typically most prominent in leads V_2 and V_3.

- Prominent U wave: Amplitude > 1.5 mm

14. Pacemakers

Overview

Pacemakers are described by a four-letter code:

- First letter: Refers to the chamber(s) *PACED* (**A**trial, **V**entricular, or **D**ual).

- Second letter: Refers to the chamber *SENSED* (**A**, **V**, or **D**).

- Third letter: Refers to the pacemaker *MODE* (**I**nhibited, **T**riggered, or **D**ual).

- Fourth letter: Refers to the presence (**R**) or absence (no letter) of *RATE RESPONSIVENESS*. Rate-responsive (or rate-adaptive) pacemakers can vary their rate of pacing in response to sensed motion or physiologic alternations (e.g., QT interval, temperature) produced by exercise.

  For example, a **VVIR** pacemaker PACES the **V**entricle, SENSES the **V**entricle, is **I**NHIBITED by a sensed QRS complex, and is **R**ate responsive. A DDD pacemaker PACES and SENSES the atria and ventricle; the DUAL MODE indicates that sensed atrial activity will inhibit atrial output and trigger a ventricular output after a designated AV interval, and that sensed ventricular activity will inhibit ventricular output and trigger a ventricular output.

- Typical single-chamber pacemakers include VVI and AAI.
- Typical dual-chamber pacemakers include DVI and DDD.

Approach to Pacemaker Evaluation

Step 1: Assess underlying rhythm. Determine if the rhythm is 100% paced or if there is a nonpaced intrinsic rhythm with a pacemaker functioning in demand mode.

- 100% ventricular paced

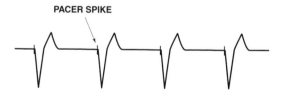

PACER SPIKE

- Ventricular pacing in *demand mode* (inconstant ventricular pacing from output inhibition by intrinsic sinus rhythm)

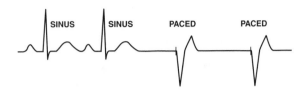

Step 2: Determine the chamber(s) PACED. Determine the relationship of pacing spikes to P waves and QRS complexes: A spike preceding the P wave typically represents atrial pacing; a spike preceding the QRS complex typically represents ventricular pacing.

- Atrial (A)-paced beat

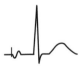

- Ventricular (V)-paced beat

- Atrial (A)- and ventricular (V)-paced beat

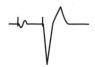

Step 3: Determine timing intervals from two consecutively paced beats.

- For atrial pacing, determine the A-A interval.

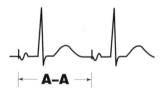

- For ventricular pacing, determine the V-V interval.

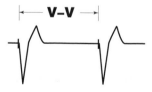

- For dual-chamber pacing, determine the A-V and V-A intervals.

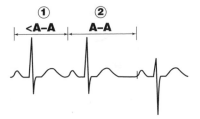

Step 4: Determine the chamber(s) SENSED.

- **Atrial pacemaker:** Proper atrial sensing is present when intrinsic atrial activation (native P wave) is followed by (1) a native P wave that occurs at an interval less than the A-A interval or (2) an atrial-paced beat that occurs after an interval equal to the A-A interval.

- **Ventricular pacemaker:** Proper ventricular sensing is present when intrinsic ventricular activation (native QRS complex) is always followed by (1) a native QRS complex that occurs at an interval less than the V-V interval or (2) a ventricular-paced beat that occurs after an interval equal to the V-V interval.

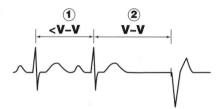

- **Dual-chamber pacemaker:**
  - *Atrial sensing* is evident when intrinsic atrial activation (native P wave) is always followed by (1) a native QRS complex that occurs at an interval less than the A-V interval or (2) a ventricular-paced beat that occurs at an interval equal to the A-V interval.

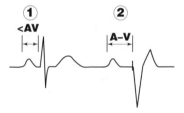

▸ *Ventricular sensing* is evident when intrinsic ventricular activation (native QRS complex) is always followed by (1) a native P wave that occurs at an interval
less than the V-A interval or (2) an atrial-paced beat
that occurs at an interval equal to the V-A interval.

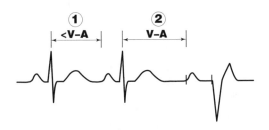

Step 5: Determine the sequence of complexes representing
normal pacing function. Keep in mind that single-chamber
pacing on the surface ECG does not exclude the possibility
that a dual-chamber pacemaker is present—ventricular-paced
beats may be due to a single-chamber ventricular pacemaker
or a dual-chamber pacemaker in which ventricular spikes are
timed to follow P waves (DDD pacemaker) (Table 2).

Table 2		
Pacing mode	**Atrial pacing spike**	**Ventricular pacing spike**
Atrial pacing	+	–
Ventricular pacing	–	+
Dual-chamber pacing	+	+
(DDD) pacing	+ – –	– + –
+ Pacing spike present on surface ECG – Pacing spike absent on surface ECG		

Step 6: Look for pacemaker malfunction.

- **Failure to capture** (see item 93, Section 3): Are any pacing spikes not followed by a depolarization?

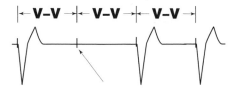

- **Sensing Abnormalities:**
  - **Undersensing:** Based on timing intervals, are there pacing spikes that should have been inhibited by a native P wave or QRS complex but were not? This results in a paced beat that appears *earlier* than expected. ***Example***: For ventricular pacing, undersensing is evident when a native QRS complex is followed by a ventricular-paced beat at an interval < V-V interval.

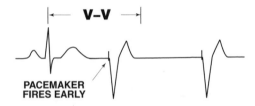

  - **Oversensing:** Based on timing intervals, are there pacing spikes that should have been initiated after a native P wave or QRS complex but were not? This results in a paced beat that appears *later* than expected. For ventricular pacing, oversensing occurs when a native QRS is followed by a ventricular-paced beat at an interval much greater than the V-V interval.

    - Oversensing of the T wave, in which the T wave is sensed as (mistaken for) a QRS complex:

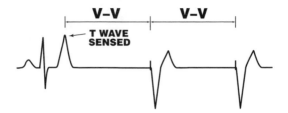

- Oversensing of muscle contractions (myopotential inhibition), in which a myopotential is sensed as (mistaken for) a QRS complex:

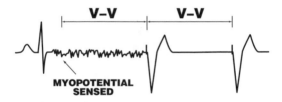

- **Other Causes of Pacemaker Malfunction:** Less common types of pacemaker malfunction include pacemaker not firing, pacemaker slowing, and pacemaker-mediated tachycardia.

— Section 2 —

ECG DIFFERENTIAL DIAGNOSIS

....

Throughout this section, item numbers noted within parentheses correspond to criteria in Section 3.

1. P Wave

Lead I

Inverted P wave

- Ectopic atrial premature beat (item 13) or rhythm (items 15, 17)
- AV junctional/ventricular premature complex (items 20, 23) or rhythm with retrograde atrial activation
- Dextrocardia (item 80): Inverted P-QRS-T in leads I and aVL with *reverse* R-wave progression in the precordial leads
- Reversal of right and left arm leads (item 3): Inverted P-QRS-T in leads I and aVL with *normal* R-wave progression in the precordial leads

Lead II

Tall peaked P wave

- Right atrial abnormality/enlargement (item 5)
- Biatrial abnormality

Bifid P wave with peak-to-peak interval < 0.03 second

- Normal

Bifid P wave with peak-to-peak interval > 0.03 second and P-wave duration > 0.12 second

- Left atrial abnormality/enlargement (item 6)

Inverted P wave

- Ectopic atrial premature beat (item 13) or rhythm (items 15, 17)
- AV junctional/ventricular premature complex (items 20, 23) or rhythm with retrograde atrial activation

Sawtooth regular P waves

- Atrial flutter (item 18)
- Artifact due to tremor (e.g., Parkinson disease, shivering) (item 4)

Irregularly irregular baseline

- Atrial fibrillation (item 19)
- Artifact due to tremor (item 4)
- Multifocal atrial tachycardia (item 16)

Multiple P-wave morphologies

- Wandering atrial pacemaker (rate < 100 bpm)
- Multifocal atrial tachycardia (rate > 100 bpm) (item 16)
- Sinus or atrial rhythm with multiple atrial premature complexes

Lead V₁

Tall upright P wave

- Right atrial abnormality/enlargement (item 5)

Deep inverted P waves

- Left atrial abnormality/enlargement (item 6)

Dome and dart P wave

- Ectopic atrial rhythm (item 15)

No P Waves

P waves present but hidden

- Ectopic atrial rhythm or APCs (P waves hidden in preceding T wave)
- Junctional rhythm or SVT (P wave buried in QRS)
- Supraventricular rhythm with marked first-degree AV block (P wave hidden in preceding T wave)

P waves not present

- Sinoventricular conduction due to hyperkalemia (item 74)
- Marked sinoatrial exit block or sinus bradycardia with junctional or ventricular rhythm (escape or accelerated)
- Sinus pause or arrest (item 11)

2. PR Interval

Prolonged (> 0.20 second) PR interval

- First-degree AV block (item 29)
- Complete heart block (item 33): PR interval varies, has no constant relationship to the QRS, and may intermittently exceed 0.20 second
- Supraventricular or junctional rhythm with retrograde atrial activation: P wave inverted in lead II
- Atrial premature complex (item 13)

Short (< 0.12 second) PR interval

- Short PR with sinus rhythm and normal QRS
- Wolff-Parkinson-White pattern (item 34): Delta wave, wide QRS, ST-T changes in a direction opposite to main deflection of QRS
- Low ectopic atrial rhythm: PR interval usually > 0.11 second; P wave inverted in lead II
- Ectopic junctional beat or rhythm with retrograde atrial activation: PR interval usually < 0.11 second; P wave inverted in lead II

3. PR Segment

PR-segment depression

- Normals: < 0.8 mm
- Pericarditis (item 84)
- Pseudodepression due to atrial flutter (item 18) or Parkinsonian tremor (item 4)
- Atrial infarction: Reciprocal elevation in opposite leads; inferior MI usually evident

PR-segment elevation

- Normals: < 0.5 mm
- Pericarditis (item 84): Lead aVR only
- Atrial infarction: Reciprocal depression in opposite leads

4. QRS Duration

Increased QRS duration 0.10 to < 0.12 second

- Left anterior fascicular block (item 45)
- Left posterior fascicular block (item 46)
- Incomplete LBBB (item 48)
- Incomplete RBBB (item 44)
- Nonspecific IVCD (item 49)
- LVH (item 40)
- RVH (item 41)
- Supraventricular beat or rhythm with aberrant intraventricular conduction (item 50)
- Fusion beats
- Wolff-Parkinson-White pattern (item 34)
- VPCs originating near the bundle of His (i.e., high in the interventricular septum)

Increased QRS duration > 0.12 second

- RBBB (item 43)
- LBBB (item 47)
- Supraventricular beat or rhythm with aberrant intraventricular conduction (item 50)
- Fusion beats
- Wolff-Parkinson-White pattern (item 34)
- Ventricular premature complexes (item 23)
- Ventricular rhythm (items 24–27)
- Nonspecific IVCD (item 49)
- Paced beat

5. QRS Amplitude

Low-voltage QRS

- Chronic lung disease (item 81)
- Pericardial effusion (item 83)
- Myxedema (item 87)
- Obesity
- Pleural effusion
- Restrictive or infiltrative cardiomyopathy
- Diffuse coronary artery disease

Tall QRS

- LVH (item 40)
- Hypertrophic cardiomyopathy (item 85)
- LBBB (item 47)
- Wolff-Parkinson-White pattern (item 34)
- Normal persons with thin body habitus

Prominent R wave in lead V_1

- RVH (item 41)
- Posterior wall MI (items 59, 60)
- Incorrect lead placement: Electrode for lead V_1 placed in 3rd instead of 4th intercostal space
- Skeletal deformities (e.g., pectus excavatum)
- RBBB (item 43)
- Wolff-Parkinson-White pattern (item 34)
- Duchenne's muscular dystrophy

Alternation in QRS amplitude
- Electrical alternans (item 38)

6. QRS Axis

Left axis deviation
- Left anterior fascicular block (if axis > −45°, item 45)
- Inferior wall MI (items 57, 58)
- LBBB (item 47)
- LVH (item 40)
- Ostium primum ASD (item 79)
- Chronic lung disease (item 81)
- Hyperkalemia (item 74)

Right axis deviation
- RVH (item 41)
- Vertical heart
- Chronic lung disease (item 81)
- Pulmonary embolus (item 82)
- Left posterior fascicular block (item 46)
- Lateral wall MI (items 55, 56)
- Dextrocardia (item 80)
- Lead reversal (item 3)
- Ostium secundum ASD (item 78)

7. Q Wave

Q-wave myocardial infarction (see items 51–60)

- Anterolateral MI: Abnormal Q waves in leads V_4–V_6
- Anterior MI: Abnormal Q waves in at least two consecutive leads in V_2–V_4
- Anteroseptal MI: Abnormal Q waves in leads V_1–V_3 (and sometimes V_4)
- Lateral MI: Abnormal Q waves in leads I and aVL
- Inferior MI: Abnormal Q waves in at least two of leads II, III, and aVF

Pseudoinfarcts (Q waves in absence of MI)

- Wolff-Parkinson-White pattern (item 34): Negative delta waves mimic Q waves.
- Hypertrophic cardiomyopathy (item 85): Q waves in I, aVL, V_4–V_6 due to septal hypertrophy.
- LVH (item 40): Poor R-wave progression, at times with ST elevation in V_1–V_3, can mimic anteroseptal MI. Inferior Q waves may be present and can mimic inferior MI.
- LBBB (item 47): QS pattern in V_1–V_4 mimics anteroseptal MI. Less commonly, Q waves in III and aVF mimic inferior MI.
- RVH (item 41)
- Left anterior fascicular block (item 45)
- Chronic lung disease (item 81): Q waves appear in inferior and/or right and mid-precordial leads.

Section 2 ECG Differential Diagnosis

- Amyloid, sarcoid, and other infiltrative cardiomyopathic diseases: Electrically active tissue is replaced by inert substance.
- Cardiomyopathy
- Chest deformity (e.g., pectus excavatum)
- Pulmonary embolus (item 82): Q wave in lead III and sometimes aVF, but Q waves in II are rare.
- Myocarditis
- Myocardial tumors
- Hyperkalemia (item 74)
- Pneumothorax: QS complex in right precordial leads
- Pancreatitis
- Lead reversal (item 3)
- Corrected transposition
- Muscular dystrophy
- Mitral valve prolapse: Rare Q wave in III and aVF
- Myocardial contusion: Q waves in areas of intramyocardial hemorrhage and edema
- Left/right atrial enlargement: Prominent atrial repolarization wave (Ta) can depress the PR segment and mimic Q waves.
- Atrial flutter (item 18): Flutter waves may deform the PR segment and simulate Q waves.
- Dextrocardia (item 80)

8. R-Wave Progression (Precordial Leads)

Early R-wave progression (tall R wave in V_1, V_2; R/S > 1)
- RVH (item 41)
- Posterior MI (items 59, 60)
- RBBB (item 43)
- Wolff-Parkinson-White pattern (item 34)
- Normals
- Duchenne muscular dystrophy

Poor R-wave progression (first precordial lead where R-wave amplitude $\geq$ S-wave amplitude = V_5 or V_6)
- Normals (abnormal lead placement)
- Anterior or anteroseptal MI (items 53, 54)
- Dilated or hypertrophic cardiomyopathy
- LVH (item 40)
- Chronic lung disease (item 81)
- Cor pulmonale (item 82)
- RVH (item 41)
- Left anterior fascicular block (item 45)

Reverse R-wave progression (decreasing R-wave amplitude across precordial leads)
- Anterior MI (items 53, 54)
- Dextrocardia (item 80)

9. QRS Morphology

Initial slurring of R wave (delta wave)
- Wolff-Parkinson-White pattern (item 34)

Terminal notching (of R or S wave)
- Hypothermia (Osborne wave, item 88)
- Early repolarization (item 61)
- Pacemaker spike (failure to sense, item 94)
- Atrial flutter (item 18): Flutter waves may be superimposed on QRS.
- Arrhythmogenic Right Ventricular Dysplasia/ Cardiomyopathy (Epsilon wave)

10. ST Segment

ST-segment elevation
- Myocardial injury (item 65): Convex upward ST elevation localized to a *few* leads and terminates with an inverted T (unless hyperacute-peaked T wave). Reciprocal ST depression evident in other leads. Q waves frequently present. ST and T wave changes *evolve*, and T wave becomes inverted *before* ST segment returns to baseline.
- Acute pericarditis (item 84): Widespread ST elevation (leads I–III, aVF, V_3–V_6) *without reciprocal* ST depression in other leads except aVR. No Q wave. PR-segment depression is sometimes present. ST-T–wave changes

evolve; T wave often becomes inverted *after* ST segment returns to baseline. Note: Pericarditis (and ST elevation) may be focal.

- Ventricular aneurysm: ST elevation usually with deep Q wave or QS in same leads; ST and T-wave changes persist and are *stable* over a long period of time.

- Early repolarization (item 61): Concave upward ST elevation that ends with an upward T wave, with notching on the downstroke of the R wave. T waves are usually large and symmetrical. ST-T–wave changes are *stable* over a long time period.

- LVH (item 40)

- Bundle branch block (items 43, 47)

- Central nervous system disorder (item 86)

- Apical hypertrophic cardiomyopathy (item 85)

- Hyperkalemia (item 74)

- Acute cor pulmonale (item 82)

- Myocarditis

- Myocardial tumor

ST-segment depression

- Myocardial ischemia (item 64): horizontal or downsloping

- Repolarization changes secondary to ventricular hypertrophy (item 67) or bundle branch block (items 43, 47)

- Digitalis effect (item 70)

- Pseudodepression due to superimposition of atrial flutter waves or prominent atrial repolarization wave (as seen with atrial enlargement, pericarditis, atrial infarction) on the ST segment

- Central nervous system disorder (item 86)
- Hypokalemia (item 75)
- Antiarrhythmic drug effect (item 72)
- Mitral valve prolapse

Nonspecific ST-segment changes
- Organic heart disease
- Drugs (e.g., quinidine)
- Electrolyte disorders (e.g., hypokalemia, item 75)
- Hyperventilation
- Myxedema (item 87)
- Stress
- Pancreatitis
- Pericarditis (item 84)
- Central nervous system disorder (item 86)
- LVH (item 40)
- RVH (item 41)
- Bundle branch block (items 43, 44, 47, 48)
- Healthy adults (normal variant) (item 2)

11. T Wave

Tall peaked T waves
- Hyperacute MI
- Angina pectoris

- Normal variant (item 2): Usually affects mid-precordial leads.
- Hyperkalemia (item 74): More common when the rise in serum potassium is acute.
- Intracranial bleeding (item 86)
- LVH (item 40)
- RVH (item 41)
- LBBB (item 47)
- Superimposed P wave from APC, sinus rhythm with marked first-degree AV block, complete heart block, etc.
- Anemia

Deeply inverted T waves
- Myocardial ischemia (item 64)
- LVH (items 40, 67)
- RVH (items 41, 67)
- Central nervous system disorder (item 86)
- Wolff-Parkinson-White pattern (item 34)

Nonspecific T waves
- Persistent juvenile pattern: T-wave inversion in V_1–V_3 in young adults
- Organic heart disease
- Drugs (e.g., quinidine)
- Electrolyte disorders (e.g., hypokalemia, item 75)
- Hyperventilation
- Myxedema (item 87)
- Stress

- Pancreatitis
- Pericarditis (item 84)
- Central nervous system disorder (item 86)
- LVH (item 40)
- RVH (item 41)
- Bundle branch block (items 43, 44, 47, 48)
- Healthy adults (normal variant) (item 2)

12. QT Interval

Long QT interval

- **Acquired conditions**
  - Drugs (quinidine, procainamide, disopyramide, amiodarone, sotalol, dofetilide, azimilide, phenothiazines, tricyclics, lithium)
  - Hypomagnesemia
  - Hypocalcemia (item 77)
  - Hypokalemia (item 75)
  - Marked bradyarrhythmias
  - Intracranial hemorrhage (item 86)
  - Myocarditis
  - Mitral valve prolapse
  - Myxedema (item 87)
  - Hypothermia (item 88)
  - Liquid protein diets
- **Congenital disorders**

- ‣ Romano-Ward syndrome (normal hearing)
- ‣ Jervell and Lange-Nielsen syndrome (deafness)
- ‣ Other sodium and potassium channel defects

Short QT interval
- Hypercalcemia (item 76)
- Hyperkalemia (item 74)
- Digitalis effect (item 70)
- Acidosis
- Vagal stimulation
- Hyperthyroidism
- Hyperthermia

13. U Wave

Prominent U wave
- Hypokalemia (item 75)
- Bradyarrhythmias
- Hypothermia (item 88)
- LVH (item 40)
- Coronary artery disease
- Drugs (digitalis, quinidine, amiodarone, isoproterenol)

Inverted U wave
- LVH (item 40)
- Severe RVH (item 41)
- Myocardial ischemia

14. P-P Pause > 2.0 Seconds

- Sinus pause or arrest (item 11): Due to transient failure of impulse formation at the SA node. Sinus rhythm resumes at a P-P interval that is not a multiple of the basic sinus P-P interval.

- Sinus arrhythmia (item 8): Phasic gradual change in P-P interval.

- Second-degree sinoatrial exit block, Mobitz I (Wencke-bach) (item 12): Progressive shortening of P-P interval until a P wave fails to appear.

- Second-degree sinoatrial exit block, Mobitz II (item 12): Pause followed by resumption of sinus rhythm at a P-P interval that is a multiple (e.g., 2×, 3×, etc.) of the basic sinus rhythm.

- Third-degree sinoatrial exit block (item 12): Complete failure of sinoatrial conduction; cannot be differentiated from complete sinus arrest on surface ECG.

- Abrupt change in autonomic tone.

- "Pseudo" sinus pause due to nonconducted APCs (item 13): P wave appears to be absent but is actually buried in the T wave—look for subtle deformity of the T wave just preceding the pause to detect nonconducted APCs.

15. Group Beating

- Mobitz type I, second-degree AV block (item 30)
- Mobitz type II, second-degree AV block (item 31)
- Blocked APCs (item 13)
- Concealed His-bundle depolarizations

Section 3 ECG Criteria

General Features

1. NORMAL ECG (NO ABNORMALITIES OF RATE, RHYTHM, AXIS, OR P-QRS-T)

P wavek

- *Duration*: 0.08–0.11 second
- *Axis*: 0–75°
- *Morphology*: Upright in I, II; upright or inverted in aVF; inverted or biphasic in III, aVL, V_1, V_2; small notching may be present.
- *Amplitude*: Limb leads < 2.5 mm; V_1: positive deflection < 1.5 mm and negative deflection < 1 mm

PR interval

- *Duration*: 0.12–0.20 second
- *PR segment*: Usually isoelectric; may be displaced in a direction opposite to the P wave; elevation is usually < 0.5 mm; depression is typically < 0.8 mm.

QRS complex

- *Duration*: 0.06–0.10 second
- *Axis*: $-30°$ to $+105°$
- *Transition zone (precordial leads with equal positive and negative deflection)*: V_2–V_4
- *Q wave*: Small Q waves (duration < 0.04 second and amplitude < 2 mm) are common in most leads except aVR, V_1, and V_2.
- *Onset of intrinsicoid deflection (beginning of QRS to peak of R wave)*: Right precordial leads < 0.035 second; left precordial leads < 0.045 second

ST segment

- Usually isoelectric. In limb leads, may vary from 0.5 mm below to 1 mm above baseline; in V_2–V_3 (sometimes V_4), up to 3 mm concave upward elevation in precordial leads may be seen in young adults (early repolarization, item 61), but is usually < 2 mm if over age 40 years; in V_5–V_6, concave upward elevation more than 1 mm is uncommon.

T wave

- *Morphology*: Upright in I, II, V_3–V_6; inverted in aVR, V_1; may be upright, flat, or biphasic in III, aVL, aVF, V_1, V_2; T-wave inversion may be present in V_1–V_3 in healthy young adults (juvenile T waves, item 62).
- *Amplitude*: Usually < 6 mm in limb leads and < 10 mm in precordial leads

QT interval

- Corrected QT (QT interval divided by the square root of the R-R interval) = 0.30–0.44 second; varies inversely with heart rate

U wave

- *Morphology*: Upright in all leads except aVR
- *Amplitude*: 5–25% the height of the T wave (usually < 1.5 mm)

2. BORDERLINE NORMAL ECG OR NORMAL VARIANT

- Early repolarization (item 61)
- Juvenile T waves (item 62)
- S wave in leads I, II, and III ($S_1S_2S_3$ pattern). *Note*: Present in up to 20% of healthy young adults.
- RSR′ or rSr′ in lead V_1 with QRS duration < 0.10 second, r-wave amplitude < 7 mm, and r′ amplitude smaller than r or S waves. *Note*: Seen in 2% of normals, but can also be seen in:
  - ▸ RVH (item 41)

- ‣ Posterior MI (items 59, 60)
- ‣ Skeletal deformities (pectus excavatum, straight back syndrome)
- ‣ High electrode placement of V_1 (in 3rd intercostal space instead of 4th)
- Tall P waves
- Notched P waves of normal duration

Note: Hyperventilation may cause prolonged PR, sinus tachycardia, and ST depression ± T-wave inversion (usually seen in inferior leads).

Note: Large food intake may cause ST depression and/or T-wave inversion, especially after a high carbohydrate meal.

3. INCORRECT ELECTRODE PLACEMENT

Limb lead reversal:

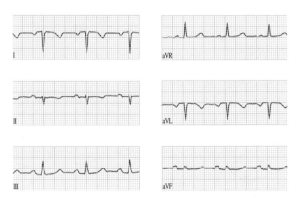

- Reversal of right and left arm leads
  - Resultant ECG mimics dextrocardia in limb leads with inversion of the P-QRS-T in leads I and aVL
  - Leads II and III transposed
  - Leads aVR and aVL transposed

  Note: To distinguish between these conditions, look at precordial leads: dextrocardia shows reverse R-wave progression (with gradual loss of R-wave voltage from V_1 to V_6); limb lead reversal shows normal R-wave progress
- Reversal of left arm and left leg leads
  - Leads I and II transposed
  - Leads aVF and aVL transposed
  - Lead III inverted
- Reversal of right arm and left leg leads
  - Leads I, II, and III inverted
  - Leads aVR and aVF transposed

Precordial lead reversal: Typically manifests as an unexplained decrease in R-wave voltage in two consecutive leads (e.g., V_1, V_2) with a return to normal R-wave progression on the following leads.

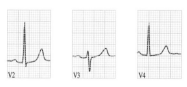

4. ARTIFACT

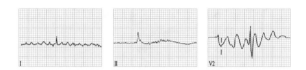

- **AC electrical interference** (60 cycles per second): Due to an unstable or dry electrode, poor grounding of the ECG machine, or excessive current leak from an ECG machine too close to other electronic equipment. Rapid sine-wave changes make assessment of P waves and ST-segment shifts unreliable.

- **Wandering baseline:** Due to an unstable electrode, deep respirations, or uncooperative patient. Evaluation of P waves, QRS voltage, and ST-segment shifts are unreliable.

- **Skeletal muscle fasciculations** (e.g., shivering, anxiety with muscle tension)

- Commonly due to **tremor** (most prominent in limb leads)
  - ‣ Parkinsonian tremor simulates atrial flutter with a rate of ~ 300 per minute (4–6 cycles per second)
  - ‣ Physiologic tremor rate is 500 per minute (7–9 per second)

- **Poor standardization:** 1 mV signal is not recorded, underdamped, or overdamped; ECG recorded at half-standard or double-standard. Voltages may be inaccurate.

- **ECG recorded at double-speed or half-speed**

- **Rapid arm motion** or lead movement (e.g., brushing teeth or hair): Can simulate VPCs or ventricular tachycardia; often mistaken for ventricular tachycardia on telemetry or Holter monitoring.

- **Cautery:** Pronounced baseline interference
- **IV infusion pump:** May give appearance of rapid P waves

P-Wave Abnormalities

5. RIGHT ATRIAL ABNORMALITY/ENLARGEMENT

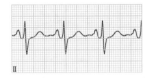

- Tall upright P wave:
  - \> 2.5 mm in leads II, III, and aVF (P pulmonale), *or*
  - \> 1.5 mm in leads V_1 or V_2
- P-wave axis shifted rightward (i.e., axis ≥ 70°)

  Note: In up to 30% of cases, P pulmonale may actually represent left atrial enlargement. Suspect this possibility when left atrial abnormality/enlargement (item 6) is present in lead V_1.

  Note: Prominent atrial repolarization waves (Ta) can mimic Q waves and ST depression by deforming the PR and ST segments, respectively.

  Note: P pulmonale can be seen in:
  - COPD with or without cor pulmonale (item 81)
  - Pulmonary hypertension

- ‣ Congenital heart disease (such as pulmonic stenosis, tetralogy of Fallot, tricuspid atresia, Eisenmenger physiology)
- ‣ Pulmonary embolus (usually transient) (item 82)
- ‣ Normal variant in patients with a thin body habitus and/or vertical heart

6. LEFT ATRIAL ABNORMALITY/ENLARGEMENT

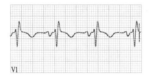

- Terminal negative portion of the P wave in lead $V_1 \geq 1$ mm deep and ≥ 0.04 second in duration (i.e., one small box deep and one small box wide), *or*
- Notched P wave with a duration ≥ 0.12 second in leads II, III, or aVF (P mitrale)

   Note: Left atrial enlargement by echocardiography can exist with a normal P wave, and P mitrale may be present in the absence of left atrial enlargement.

   Note: Prominent atrial repolarization waves (Ta) can mimic Q waves and ST depression by deforming the PR and ST segments, respectively.

   Note: Mechanisms responsible for P mitrale include left atrial hypertrophy or dilation, intraatrial conduction delay, increased left atrial volume, and an acute rise in left atrial pressure.

Note: Can be seen in:

- ▸ Mitral valve disease
- ▸ Organic heart disease
- ▸ Aortic valve disease
- ▸ Heart failure
- ▸ Myocardial infarction
- ▸ Hypertension/LVH

Supraventricular Rhythms

7. SINUS RHYTHM

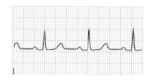

- Normal P-wave axis and morphology
- Atrial rate is 60–100 per minute and regular (P-P interval varies by < 0.16 second or < 10%).

8. SINUS ARRHYTHMIA

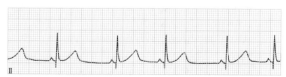

- Normal P-wave morphology and axis
- Phasic change in P-P interval (onset may sometimes occur abruptly), usually in response to the breath cycle
- Longest and shortest P-P intervals vary by > 0.16 second or 10%.

  Note: Sinus arrhythmia is a major factor in beat-to-beat heart rate variability (HRV). The presence of maintained HRV is a manifestation of active, healthy, vagal tone, and an important marker for good cardiovascular prognosis.

9. SINUS BRADYCARDIA (< 60)

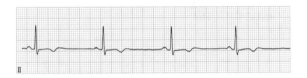

- Normal P-wave axis and morphology
- Rate < 60 per minute

  Note: If the atrial rate is < 40 per minute, think of 2:1 sinoatrial exit block (item 12)

  Note: Causes include:

  ‣ High vagal tone (normals, especially during sleep; trained athletes; Bezold-Jarisch reflex; inferior MI, pulmonary embolus)

  ‣ Myocardial infarction (usually inferior)

  ‣ Drugs (b-blockers; verapamil; diltiazem; digitalis; type IA, IB, IC antiarrhythmics; amiodarone; sotalol;

clonidine; a-methyldopa; reserpine; guanethidine; lithium)

‣ Hypothyroidism (item 87)

‣ Hypothermia (item 88)

‣ Obstructive jaundice

‣ Hyperkalemia (item 74)

‣ Increased intracranial pressure (item 86)

‣ Sick sinus syndrome (item 89)

10. SINUS TACHYCARDIA (> 100)

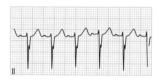

• Normal P-wave axis and morphology

• Rate > 100 per minute

   Note: P-wave amplitude often increases and PR interval often shortens with increasing heart rate (e.g., during exercise).

   Note: Causes include:

   ‣ Physiologic response to stress (exercise, anxiety, pain, fever, hypovolemia, hypotension, anemia)

   ‣ Thyrotoxicosis

   ‣ Myocardial ischemia/infarction

   ‣ Heart failure

   ‣ Myocarditis

- ▸ Pulmonary embolus (item 82)
- ▸ Pheochromocytoma
- ▸ AV fistula
- ▸ Drugs (caffeine, alcohol, nicotine, cocaine, amphetamines, albuterol and other beta-agonists, endogenous catecholamines, hydralazine, exogenous thyroid, atropine, aminophylline)

11. SINUS PAUSE OR ARREST

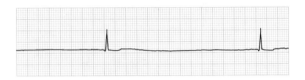

- • P-P interval (pause) greater than 1.6–2.0 seconds
- • Sinus pause is *not* a multiple of the basic sinus P-P interval

    Note: If sinus pause is a multiple of the basic P-P interval, consider sinoatrial exit block (item 12).

    Note: Sinus pauses must be differentiated from:

    - ▸ *Sinus arrhythmia* (item 8): Phasic, gradual change in P-P interval
    - ▸ *Second-degree sinoatrial block, Mobitz I* (Wenckebach) (item 12): Progressive shortening of P-P interval until a P wave fails to appear
    - ▸ *Second-degree sinoatrial block, Mobitz II* (item 12): Sinus pause is a multiple (e.g., 2×, 3×, etc.) of the basic sinus rhythm (P-P interval)
    - ▸ *Abrupt change in autonomic tone* (e.g., vagal reaction)

▸ *"Pseudo" sinus pause* due to nonconducted atrial pre-mature complexes (APC) (item 13): P wave appears to be absent but is actually buried in the T wave—look for subtle deformity of the T wave at the beginning of the pause to detect nonconducted APCs.

Note: Complete failure of sinoatrial conduction (third-degree sinoatrial block, item 12) cannot be differentiated from complete sinus arrest on surface ECG.

Note: Sinus pause/arrest is due to transient failure of impulse formation at the SA node. Etiology is the same as sinoatrial exit block (item 12).

12. SINOATRIAL EXIT BLOCK

Second-degree: Some sinus impulses fail to capture the atria, resulting in the intermittent absence of a P wave. Often a component of the sick sinus syndrome (item 89).

• *Type I (Mobitz I) sinoatrial exit block:*

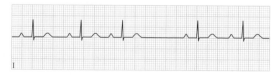

▸ P-wave morphology and axis consistent with a sinus node origin
▸ "Group beating" with:
  (1) Shortening of P-P interval up to pause
  (2) Constant PR interval
  (3) P-P pause < 2× the normal P-P interval

- *Type II (Mobitz II) sinoatrial exit block:*

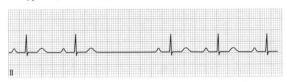

> Constant P-P interval followed by a pause that is a multiple (e.g., 2×, 3×, etc.) of the normal P-P interval.

> The pause may be slightly less than twice the normal P-P interval (usually within 0.10 second).

Note: Causes include:

> Drugs (digitalis, quinidine, flecainide, propafenone, procainamide)

> Hyperkalemia (item 74)

> Sinus node dysfunction

> Organic heart disease

> Myocardial infarction

> Vagal stimulation

Note: First-degree sinoatrial exit block (conduction of sinus impulses to the atrium is delayed, but 1:1 response is maintained) is not detectable on surface ECG, and third-degree sinoatrial exit block (complete failure of sinoatrial conduction) cannot be differentiated from complete sinus arrest (item 11).

13. ATRIAL PREMATURE COMPLEXES

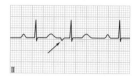

- P wave that is abnormal in configuration and premature relative to the normal P-P interval
- QRS complex is usually similar in morphology to the QRS complex present during sinus rhythm. Exceptions include:
  - *Aberrantly conducted APCs*: QRS may be wide and bizarre; more likely to occur with very premature APCs. QRS morphology is most often RBBB pattern (due to the longer refractory period of the right bundle compared to the left bundle), but can be LBBB pattern or variable.
  - *Blocked APCs:* Very premature P wave not followed by a QRS complex. P waves are often hidden in the preceding T wave; look for a deformed T wave immediately after the first QRS of the R-R pause to identify the presence of a nonconducted atrial premature complex.
- The PR interval may be normal, increased, or decreased.
- The postextrasystolic pause is usually *noncompensatory* (i.e., the interval from the preceding normal P wave to the normal P wave following the APC is less than two normal P-P intervals). However, an interpolated APC or a compensatory pause may be evident when sinoatrial (SA) "entrance block" is present and the SA node is not reset.

Note: Can be seen in normals, fatigue, stress, smoking, drugs (including caffeine and alcohol), organic heart disease, cor pulmonale.

14. ATRIAL PARASYSTOLE

- Frequent atrial premature complexes of similar morphology that "march through" the tracing independent of the underlying sinus rhythm.

- Interectopic intervals are a multiple (2×, 3×, etc.) of the shortest interectopic interval (since the parasystolic focus fires at a regular rate and inscribes a P wave whenever the atria are not refractory).

- Resultant ectopic atrial complex varies in relationship to the preceding sinus beats (i.e., nonfixed coupling).

Note: Exit block from a parasystolic focus may occur and result in absence of an atrial ectopic beat when it would otherwise be expected to occur.

Note: Atrial parasystole is due to the presence of an ectopic atrial focus that activates the atria independent of the basic sinus rhythm, and is protected from depolarization by an entrance block. The atrial focus fires at a regular cycle length and results in an ectopic atrial beat that bears no constant relationship (nonfixed coupling) to the previous sinus beat.

Note: Think of atrial parasystole in the presence of atrial premature complexes of similar morphology with nonfixed coupling.

15. ATRIAL TACHYCARDIA

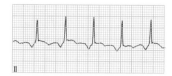

- Three or more consecutive ectopic atrial beats (nonsinus P waves) at an atrial rate of 100–240 per minute.

- P wave may precede, be buried in (sometimes not visualized), or immediately follow the QRS complex.

- QRS complex follows each P wave unless second- or third-degree AV block is present. Atrial tachycardia with block may be confused with atrial flutter. Atrial tachycardia with block has a distinct isoelectric baseline between P waves; atrial flutter does not (except occasionally in lead V_1). Atrial tachycardia with block is secondary to digitalis toxicity (item 71) in 75% and organic heart disease in 25%.

- QRS morphology is usually narrow and resembles QRS morphology during sinus rhythm, but can be wide (if underlying bundle branch block or aberrancy).

Note: Automatic atrial tachycardia and intraatrial reentrant tachycardia account for 10% of SVTs. Carotid sinus massage produces AV block but does not terminate the tachycardia. Nonsustained form is common in normals; the sustained form is more common in organic heart disease.

16. ATRIAL TACHYCARDIA, MULTIFOCAL

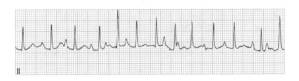

- Atrial rate > 100 per minute
- P waves with ≥ 3 morphologies (each originating from a separate atrial focus)
- Varying P-P and PR intervals
- P waves may be blocked (i.e., not followed by a QRS complex), or may be conducted with a narrow or wide (if underlying bundle branch block or aberrancy) QRS complex.

   Note: Multifocal atrial tachycardia may be confused with:

   ‣ *Sinus tachycardia with multifocal APCs*, which demonstrates one dominant atrial pacemaker (i.e., the sinus node). In contrast, in multifocal atrial tachycardia, *no* dominant atrial pacemaker (i.e., no dominant P-wave morphology) is present.

   ‣ *Atrial fibrillation/flutter,* in which there is lack of an isoelectric baseline. In contrast, multifocal atrial tachycardia demonstrates a distinct isoelectric baseline and P waves.

   Note: Usually associated with some form of lung disease. Etiologies include:

   ‣ COPD/pneumonia
   ‣ Cor pulmonale

> ‣ Aminophylline therapy
> ‣ Hypoxia
> ‣ Organic heart disease
> ‣ Heart failure
> ‣ Postoperative state
> ‣ Sepsis
> ‣ Pulmonary edema

17. SUPRAVENTRICULAR TACHYCARDIA, PAROXYSMAL

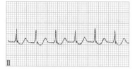

Without aberrancy

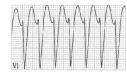

With aberrancy

- Regular rhythm
- Rate > 100 per minute
- P waves not easily identified
- QRS complex is usually narrow (but occasionally wide if underlying bundle branch block or aberrancy).
- Onset and termination of SVT is sudden, and SVT does not persist throughout the entire tracing.
- Retrograde atrial activity may be present.

  Note: If rate is approximately 150 per minute, atrial flutter with 2:1 block may be present. Look for typical "sawtooth" flutter waves in inferior leads (II, III, aVF) or V_1;

every other flutter wave may be buried in the QRS complex or ST segment.

Note: There are several different types of supraventricular tachycardias, the majority of which cannot be differentiated by surface ECG alone and may require an electrophysiology (EP) study to differentiate:

▸ *AV nodal reentrant tachycardia* accounts for 60–70% of SVTs and is usually initiated by an APC. Reentry occurs in the AV node, with antegrade conduction down the slow (α) AV nodal pathway and retrograde conduction up the fast (β) AV nodal pathway. Carotid sinus massage slows and frequently terminates tachycardia. Occurs commonly in normals. The presence of an R′ in V_1 during tachycardia that is absent during sinus rhythm suggests AV nodal reentrant tachycardia.

▸ *Atypical AV nodal reentrant tachycardia* accounts for 5–10% of AV node reentry and 2–5% of SVTs. Reentry circuit in AV node with antegrade conduction down the rapid (β) AV node pathway and retrograde conduction up the slow (α) pathway. May require an EP study to diagnose. Carotid sinus massage may terminate the tachycardia.

▸ *AV reentrant tachycardia (orthodromic SVT)* occurs with Wolff-Parkinson-White syndrome and concealed bypass tracts. The hearts are usually normal in these conditions, but WPW can be associated with Ebstein's anomaly, cardiomyopathy, or mitral valve prolapse. Usually a short RP SVT, but can have a long RP interval and be incessant if there is slow retrograde (VA) conduction. Often initiated by APCs and usually terminates suddenly with carotid sinus massage.

▸ In contrast to the other forms of atrial tachycardia, *sinus node reentrant tachycardia* manifests *sinus* P waves and is indistinguishable from sinus tachycardia. It involves reentry in or around the sinus node and accounts for < 5% of SVTs. Carotid sinus massage produces AV block but does not terminate the tachycardia. Occasionally seen in normals but more common in organic heart disease.

18. ATRIAL FLUTTER

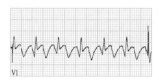

• Rapid regular atrial undulations (flutter or "F" waves) usually at a rate of 240–340 per minute

Note: Flutter rate may be faster (> 340 per minute) in children and slower (200–240 per minute) in the presence of antiarrhythmic drugs (type IA, IC, III) and/or massively dilated atria.

Note: ECG artifact due to Parkinsonian tremor (~ 4–6 cycles per second) can simulate flutter waves. Look for evidence of distinct superimposed P waves preceding each QRS complex, especially in leads I, II, or V_1.

• Typical atrial flutter morphology is usually present:

▸ Leads II, III, aVF: Inverted F waves without an iso-electric baseline ("picket-fence" or "sawtooth" appearance)

- ‣ Lead V_1: Small positive deflections usually with a distinct isoelectric baseline
- Atypical atrial flutter can exhibit upright F waves in inferior leads.
- QRS complex may be normal or wide (if underlying bundle branch block or aberrancy).
- Rate and regularity of QRS complexes depend on the AV conduction sequence: AV conduction ratio (ratio of flutter waves to QRS complexes) is usually fixed and an even number (e.g., 2:1, 4:1), but may vary.

Note: Odd-numbered conduction ratios of 1:1 and 3:1 are uncommon. Atrial flutter with 1:1 AV conduction often conducts aberrantly, resulting in a wide QRS tachycardia that may be confused with VT. In untreated patients, $\geq$ 4:1 block suggests the coexistence of AV conduction disease.

Note: Carotid sinus massage typically causes a transient increase in AV block and slowing of the ventricular response, without a change in the atrial flutter rate. At times, no effect is seen. When atrial flutter with 2:1 AV block is suspected, carotid sinus massage may unmask flutter waves and help confirm the diagnosis. Upon discontinuation of carotid sinus massage, the usual response is return to the original ventricular rate.

- Complete heart block with a junctional or ventricular escape rhythm may be present.

Note: Consider digitalis toxicity in the setting of atrial flutter with complete heart block and junctional tachycardia.

Note: Flutter waves can deform QRS, ST, and/or T to mimic intraventricular conduction delay and/or myocardial ischemia.

Note: Etiology is the same as for atrial fibrillation (item 19).

19. ATRIAL FIBRILLATION

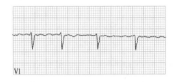

- P waves absent
- Atrial activity is totally irregular and represented by fibrillatory (f) waves of varying amplitude, duration, and morphology, causing random oscillation of the baseline.

  Note: Atrial activity is best seen in leads V_1, V_2, II, III, aVF.

- Ventricular rhythm is typically irregularly irregular.

  Note: If the R-R interval is regular, second- or third-degree AV block may be present.

  Note: Digitalis toxicity may result in regularization of the QRS due to complete heart block with junctional tachycardia.

- Ventricular rate is usually 100–180 per minute in the absence of drugs.

  Note: If the rate without AV-blocking drugs is less than 100 beats per minute, AV conduction system disease is likely to be present.

  Note: Consider **Wolff-Parkinson-White syndrome** (item 34) if the ventricular rate is > 200 per minute and the QRS is > 0.12 second. The 12-lead ECG during sinus rhythm should show a short PR interval and a wide QRS complex with initial slurring (delta wave):

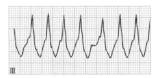

Note: Conditions mimicking atrial fibrillation include:
▸ Multifocal atrial tachycardia (item 16)
▸ Atrial flutter (item 18)
Note: Etiologies include:
▸ Mitral valve disease (especially if severe)
▸ Organic heart disease
▸ Hypertension
▸ Post-CABG (30% of patients)
▸ Myocardial infarction
▸ Thyrotoxicosis
▸ Pulmonary embolus (item 82)
▸ Postoperative state
▸ Hypoxia
▸ Chronic lung disease (e.g., emphysema) (item 81)
▸ Atrial septal defect (items 78, 79)
▸ Wolff-Parkinson-White syndrome (item 34)
▸ Sick sinus syndrome (tachy-brady syndrome) (item 89)
▸ Alcohol ("holiday heart" syndrome)
▸ Normals (lone atrial fibrillation)

Junctional Rhythms

20. AV JUNCTIONAL PREMATURE COMPLEXES

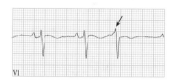

- Premature QRS complex (relative to the basic R-R interval), which may be narrow or wide (if underlying bundle branch block or aberrancy)

- The P wave may precede the QRS by ≤ 0.11 second (retrograde atrial activation), may be buried in the QRS (and not visualized), or may follow the QRS complex.

- Inverted P waves in leads II, III, and aVF and upright P waves in leads I and aVL are commonly seen due to the spread of atrial activation from near the AV node and in a superior and leftward direction (i.e., away from the inferior leads and toward the left lateral leads).

Note: The atrium may occasionally be activated by the sinus node, resulting in a normal sinus P wave. This occurs when retrograde block exists between the AV junctional focus and the atrium, or the sinus node activates the atrium before the AV junctional impulse.

Note: A constant coupling interval and noncompensatory pause are usually present.

Note: Seen in normals and organic heart disease.

21. AV JUNCTIONAL ESCAPE COMPLEXES

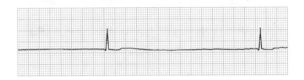

- Typically narrow QRS complex beat(s) that follow the previous conducted beat at a coupling interval corresponding to a rate of 40–60 per minute. QRS may be wide if underlying bundle branch block.
- P wave may precede (PR < 0.11 second), be buried in, or follow the QRS complex (similar to AV junctional premature complexes, item 23).
- QRS morphology is similar to the sinus or supraventricular impulse.

  Note: QRS complex occurs as a secondary phenomenon in response to decreased sinus impulse formation or conduction, high-degree AV block, or after a pause following termination of atrial tachycardia, atrial flutter, or atrial fibrillation.

22. AV JUNCTIONAL RHYTHM/TACHYCARDIA

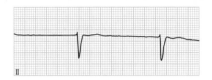

- R-R interval is usually regular.
- Heart rate is between 40–60 per minute for AV junctional rhythm and > 60 per minute for junctional tachycardia.
- P wave may precede, be buried in, or follow the QRS complex.
- QRS is usually narrow, but may be wide if underlying bundle branch block or aberrancy.
- Relationship between atrial and ventricular rates may vary:
  - If retrograde (VA) block is present, the atria remain in sinus rhythm and *AV dissociation* (item 35) will be present.
  - If retrograde atrial activation (inverted P waves in II, III, aVF) occurs, a constant QRS-P interval is usually present.

Note: Consider digitalis toxicity (item 71) if atrial fibrillation or flutter with a regular R-R interval is seen—this often represents complete heart block with junctional tachycardia.

Note: Junctional tachycardia can be seen in acute myocardial infarction (usually inferior), myocarditis, digitalis toxicity, and following open heart surgery.

Ventricular Rhythms

23. VENTRICULAR PREMATURE COMPLEXES

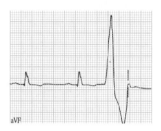

Requires all of the following:

* A wide, notched, or slurred QRS complex that is:
  ‣ Premature relative to the normal R-R interval, *and*
  ‣ Not preceded by a P wave (except when late-coupled VPCs follow a sinus P wave; in this case, the PR interval is usually ≤ 0.11 second).

  Note: QRS is almost always > 0.12 second, but VPCs originating high in the interventricular septum may have a relatively normal QRS duration.

  Note: When a VPC occurs just distal to the site of bundle branch block and near the interventricular septum, the QRS of the VPC may be narrower than the QRS of the bundle branch block.

  Note: Initial direction of the QRS is often different from the QRS during sinus rhythm.

- Secondary ST and T-wave changes in a direction opposite to the major deflection of the QRS (i.e., ST depression and T-wave inversion in leads with a dominant R wave; ST elevation and upright T wave in leads with a dominant S wave or QS complex)

- Coupling interval (relation of VPCs to the preceding QRS) may be constant or variable

  Note: Nonfixed coupling should raise the suspicion of ventricular parasystole (item 24).

- Morphology of VPCs in any given lead may be the same (uniform) or different (multiform).

  Note: Although multiform VPCs are usually multifocal in origin (i.e., originate from more than one ventricular focus), a single ventricular focus can produce VPCs of varying morphology.

  Note: Retrograde capture of atria may occur.

  Note: A full compensatory pause (P-P interval containing the VPC is twice the normal P-P interval) is usually evident, but this relationship may be altered if sinus arrhythmia is also present. A partial compensatory pause may follow a VPC when ventriculoatrial conduction penetrates and resets the sinus node. Less commonly, interpolated VPCs occur, manifesting as VPCs that are interposed between two consecutive sinus beats without disrupting the basic sinus rhythm; interpolated VPCs result in neither a partial nor a full compensatory pause.

  Note: Clues on the electrocardiogram suggestive of a ventricular (rather than atrial) origin of an ectopic beat include an initial QRS vector different from the sinus beats, QRS duration > 0.12 second, retrograde P waves (caused by retrograde conduction through the AV node), and the presence of a full compensatory pause.

Note: Seen in normals and all causes of ventricular tachycardia (item 25).

24. VENTRICULAR PARASYSTOLE

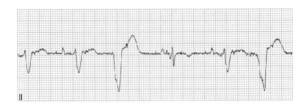

- Frequent ventricular premature complexes (VPCs) usually at a rate of 30–50 per minute with the interectopic intervals a multiple (2×, 3×, etc.) of the shortest interectopic interval present (since the parasystolic focus fires at a regular rate and inscribes a QRS complex whenever the ventricles are not refractory).

- Resultant VPCs vary in relationship to the preceding sinus or supraventricular beats (i.e., nonfixed coupling).

- VPCs typically manifest uniform morphology (which resembles a VPC, item 23) unless fusion occurs.

Note: Fusion complexes, resulting from simultaneous activation of the ventricles by atrial and parasystolic impulses, are commonly seen but are not required for the diagnosis.

Note: Exit block from a parasystolic focus may occur and result in absence of a ventricular ectopic beat when it would be expected to occur.

Note: Ventricular parasystole is due to the presence of an ectopic ventricular focus that activates the ventricles independent of the basic sinus or supraventricular rhythm, and is protected from depolarization by an entrance block. The ventricular focus fires at a regular cycle length and results in a VPC that bears no constant relationship (nonfixed coupling) to the previous sinus beat. In contrast to ventricular parasystole, uniform VPCs due to local reentry initiated by prior sinus activation of the ventricle show fixed coupling.

Note: Think of parasystole when you see ventricular premature complexes with nonfixed coupling and fusion beats.

25. VENTRICULAR TACHYCARDIA

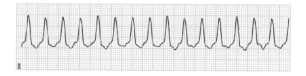

- Rapid succession of three or more ventricular premature complexes (item 23) at a rate > 100 per minute.
- R-R interval is usually regular but may be irregular.
- Abrupt onset and termination of arrhythmia is evident.
- AV dissociation (item 35) is common.

- On occasion, retrograde atrial activation, fusion complexes, and ventricular capture complexes occur.

  Note: Ventriculoatrial (VA) conduction may occur at 1:1 or may manifest variable, fixed, or complete block; ventriculoatrial Wenckebach may also occur.

  Note: In the setting of a wide QRS tachycardia, certain findings may help distinguish ventricular tachycardia from supraventricular tachycardia with aberrancy (Table 3).

  Note: Rarely, VT can present as a narrow QRS tachycardia.

  Note: Bidirectional VT is a rare type of VT in which the QRS complexes in any given lead alternate in polarity. It is most often caused by digitalis toxicity.

  Note: Seen in:
  - Organic heart disease
  - Hyperkalemia/hypokalemia (items 74, 75)
  - Hypoxia/acidosis
  - Drugs (digitalis toxicity, antiarrhythmics, phenothiazines, tricyclics, caffeine, alcohol, nicotine)
  - Mitral valve prolapse
  - Occasionally in normals

26. ACCELERATED IDIOVENTRICULAR RHYTHM

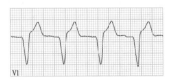

- Regular or slightly irregular ventricular (wide complex) rhythm
- Rate of 60–110 per minute
- QRS morphology similar to VPCs (item 23)
- AV dissociation (item 35), ventricular capture complexes, and fusion beats are common because of the competition between the normal sinus and ectopic ventricular rhythms.

  Note: Unlike ventricular tachycardia, AIVR is not associated with an adverse prognosis.

  Note: Seen in:
  - Myocardial ischemia
  - Following coronary reperfusion
  - Digitalis toxicity (item 71)
  - Occasionally in normals

27. VENTRICULAR ESCAPE COMPLEXES OR RHYTHM

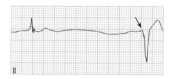

- Single beat or regular or slightly irregular ventricular rhythm
- Rate of 30–40 per minute (can be 20–50 per min)
- QRS morphology similar to VPCs (item 23)

Table 3: Origin of Wide QRS Tachycardia		
Finding	**Favors VT**	**Favors SVT with aberrancy**
QRS morphology	Similar to VPCs	Similar to sinus rhythm or APCs with aberrancy
Initiation of tachycardia	VPCs	APCs
AV dissociation present	Yes	No
Capture or fusion complexes present	Yes	No

Table 3: Origin of Wide QRS Tachycardia, continued		
Finding	**Favors VT**	**Favors SVT with aberrancy**
QRS duration when QRS is narrow during sinus rhythm	RBBB morphology (> 0.14 second); LBBB morphology (> 0.16 second)	QRS duration generally < 0.14 second
QRS deflection in precordial leads	Concordant (all positive or negative)	Discordant (some positive; some negative)
QRS axis	Left or northwest	—
RSR' in lead V$_1$	R wave taller than R'	R' taller than R wave
Lead aVR	Initial R wave; *or*, r or q > 0.04 seconds	—

Note: QRS escape complex/rhythm occurs as a secondary phenomenon in response to decreased sinus impulse formation or conduction (e.g., high vagal tone), high-degree AV block, or after the pause following termination of atrial tachycardia, atrial flutter, or atrial fibrillation.

28. VENTRICULAR FIBRILLATION

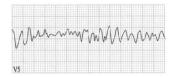

* An extremely rapid and irregular ventricular rhythm demonstrating:
  › Chaotic and irregular deflections of varying amplitude and contour
  › Absence of distinct P waves, QRS complexes, and T waves

Note: A lethal arrhythmia that can nearly always be converted into a stable rhythm when defibrillation occurs within the first minute. Successful cardioversion occurs in only 25% when delayed as little as 4–5 minutes.

AV Conduction Abnormalities

29. AV BLOCK, 1°

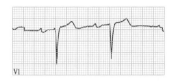

- PR interval ≥ 0.20 second (usually 0.21–0.40 second but may be as long as 0.80 second)
- Each P wave is followed by a QRS complex.

  Note: The PR interval represents the time from the onset of atrial depolarization to the onset of ventricular repolarization (i.e., conduction time from the atrium → AV node → His bundle → Purkinje system → ventricles). It does not reflect conduction from the sinus node to the atrial tissue. Therefore, a prolonged PR interval with a narrow QRS complex identifies the site of block in the AV node. If the QRS is wide, conduction delay or block typically occurs in the His-Purkinje system (although block in the AV node can manifest as a prolonged PR and wide QRS if bundle branch block or rate-dependent aberrancy is present).

  Note: Etiologies include:
  ‣ Normals
  ‣ Athletes
  ‣ High vagal tone

▸ Drugs (digitalis, quinidine, procainamide, flecainide, propafenone, amiodarone, sotalol, beta receptor blockers, verapamil, diltiazem)

▸ Acute rheumatic fever

▸ Myocarditis

▸ Congenital heart disease (atrial septal defect, patent ductus arteriosus)

30. AV BLOCK, 2°—MOBITZ TYPE I (WENCKEBACH)

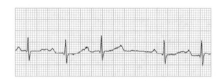

• Progressive prolongation of the PR interval and progressive shortening of the R-R interval until a P wave is blocked.

Note: The progressive shortening of the R-R interval is due to a decrease in the beat-to-beat increment of PR prolongation.

• R-R interval containing the nonconducted P wave is less than two P-P intervals.

Note: Classical Wenckebach periodicity may not always be evident, especially when sinus arrhythmia is present or an abrupt change in autonomic tone occurs.

Note: In type I block with high conduction ratios (i.e., infrequent pauses), the PR interval of the beats immediately preceding the blocked P wave may be equal to each other, suggesting type II block. In these situations, it is best to compare the PR intervals immediately before and after the blocked P wave; differences in the PR intervals suggest type I block, whereas a constant PR interval suggests type II block.

Note: Mobitz type I results in "group" or "pattern beating" due to the presence of nonconducted P waves. Other causes of group beating include:

‣ Blocked APCs

‣ Type II second-degree AV block (item 31)

‣ Concealed His-bundle depolarizations: Premature His depolarizations render the AV node refractory to subsequent sinus beats, resulting in blocked P waves and pseudo-AV block.

Note: Type I block usually occurs at the level of the AV node, resulting in a narrow QRS complex. In contrast, Mobitz type II block usually occurs within or below the bundle of His and is associated with a wide QRS complex in 80% of cases.

Note: Etiologies include:

‣ Normals

‣ Athletes

‣ Drugs (digitalis, b-blockers, verapamil, dlitiazem, clonidine, a-methyldopa, flecainide, sotalol, amiodarone, encainide, propafenone, lithium)

‣ Myocardial infarction (especially inferior)

‣ Acute rheumatic fever

‣ Myocarditis

31. AV BLOCK, 2°—MOBITZ TYPE II

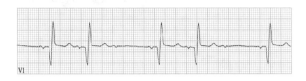

- Regular sinus or atrial rhythm with intermittent nonconducted P waves and no evidence for atrial prematurity.
- PR interval in the conducted beats is constant.
- R-R interval containing the nonconducted P wave is equal to two P-P intervals.

Note: Type II second-degree AV block usually occurs within or below the bundle of His; the QRS is wide in 80% of cases.

Note: 2:1 AV block can be Mobitz type I or II (Table 4).

Note: In type I block with high conduction rates (e.g., 10:9 conduction), the PR interval of the beats immediately preceding the blocked P wave may be equal, suggesting type II block. In these situations, it is best to compare the PR interval immediately before and after the blocked P wave; differences in the PR interval suggest type I block, whereas a constant PR interval is evidence for type II block, which is almost always due to organic heart disease.

Table 4: Features Suggesting the Mechanism of 2:1 AV Block	Mechanism	
Feature	Mobitz type I	Mobitz type II
QRS duration	Narrow	Wide
Response to maneuvers that increase heart rate and AV conduction (e.g., atropine, exercise)	Block improves	Block worsens
Response to maneuvers that reduce heart rate and AV conduction (e.g., carotid sinus massage)	Block worsens	Block improves
Develops during acute MI	Inferior MI	Anterior MI
Other	Mobitz I on another part of ECG	History of syncope

32. AV BLOCK, 2:1

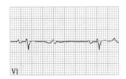

- Regular sinus or atrial rhythm with two P waves for each QRS complex (i.e., every other P wave is nonconducted)

  Note: Can be Mobitz type I or II second-degree AV block (see Table 4).

33. AV BLOCK, 3°

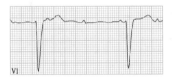

- Atrial impulses consistently fail to reach the ventricles, resulting in atrial and ventricular rhythms that are independent of each other.
- PR interval varies.
- P-P and R-R intervals are constant.
- Atrial rate is usually faster than ventricular rate.
- Ventricular rhythm is maintained by a junctional or idioventricular escape rhythm or a ventricular pacemaker.

Note: The P wave may precede, be buried within (and not visualized), or follow the QRS to deform the ST segment or T wave.

Note: Ventriculophasic sinus arrhythmia (when P-P interval containing a QRS complex is shorter than the P-P interval without a QRS complex) is present in 30–50%.

Note: Complete heart block is present when the atrial rate is faster than the ventricular escape rate (identified by the presence of nonconducted P waves when the AV node and ventricle are not refractory). In contrast, AV dissociation is usually present if the atrial rate is slower than the ventricular rate.

Note: Causes of complete heart block include:

▸ **Myocardial infarction:** 5–15% of acute myocardial infarctions are complicated by complete heart block. In inferior MI, complete heart block is usually preceded by first-degree AV block or type I second-degree AV block; it usually occurs at the level of the AV node, is typically transient (< 1 week), and is usually associated with a stable junctional escape rhythm (narrow QRS; rate ≥ 40 per minute). In anterior MI, complete heart block occurs as a result of extensive damage to the left ventricle, is typically preceded by type II second-degree AV block or bifascicular block, and is associated with mortality rates as high as 70% (due to pump failure rather than heart block, per se).

▸ **Degenerative diseases** of the conduction system (Lev disease, Lenègre disease)

▸ **Infiltrative diseases** of the myocardium (e.g., amyloid, sarcoid)

- **Digitalis toxicity:** One of the most common causes of reversible complete AV block; usually associated with a junctional escape rhythm (narrow QRS), which is often accelerated.

- **Endocarditis:** Inflammation and edema of the septum and peri-AV nodal tissues may cause conduction failure and complete heart block; PR prolongation usually precedes this event.

- **Advanced hyperkalemia** (death is usually from ventricular tachyarrhythmia)

- **Lyme disease:** Caused by a tick-borne spirochete (*Borrelia burgdorferi*), this disorder begins with a characteristic skin rash (erythema chronicum migrans) and may be followed in subsequent weeks to months by joint, cardiac, and neurological involvement. Cardiac involvement includes AV block that is partial or complete, usually occurs at the level of the AV node, and may be accompanied by syncope.

- **Others:** Myocardial contusion, acute rheumatic fever, aortic valve disease

34. WOLFF-PARKINSON-WHITE PATTERN

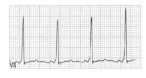

Sinus rhythm

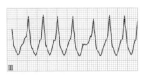

Atrial fibrillation

- Normal P-wave axis and morphology
- PR interval < 0.12 second (rarely > 0.12 second)

  Note: AV conduction over the accessory pathway (bundle of Kent) bypasses the AV node (and AV nodal conduction delay), resulting in pre-excitation of the ventricles and a short PR interval.

- Initial slurring of the QRS (delta wave), resulting in an abnormally wide QRS (> 0.12 second)

  Note: The QRS duration is ≤ 0.10 second in 30%. In these cases, the ventricles are depolarized almost entirely by the normal AV conduction system, with minimal contribution from antegrade conduction along the accessory pathway.

  Note: The widened QRS complexes represent fusion between electrical wave fronts conducted down the accessory pathway (delta wave) and the AV node. Differing degrees of pre-excitation (fusion) may be present, resulting in variability in the delta wave and QRS duration.

- Secondary ST-T–wave changes (opposite in direction to main deflection of QRS)

  Note: The PJ interval (beginning of P wave to the J point—i.e., end of QRS complex) is constant and ≤ 0.26 second. This is due to an inverse relationship between the PR interval and QRS duration—if the PR interval shortens, the QRS widens; if the PR interval lengthens, the QRS narrows.

  Note: Think WPW when atrial fibrillation or flutter is associated with a QRS that varies in width (generally wide) and has a rate > 200 per minute.

Note: Atrial fibrillation can conduct extremely rapidly, resulting in aberrant conduction and an irregular wide complex tachycardia, which resembles VT and can degenerate into VF.

Overview: Wolff-Parkinson-White syndrome (WPW) is characterized by the presence of an abnormal muscular network of specialized conduction tissue that connects the atrium to the ventricle and bypasses conduction through the AV node. It is found in 0.2–0.4% of the overall population and is more common in males and younger patients. Most patients with WPW do not have structural heart disease, although there is an increased prevalence of this disorder among patients with Ebstein anomaly (downward displacement of the tricuspid valve into the right ventricle due to anomalous attachment of the tricuspid leaflets), hypertrophic cardiomyopathy, mitral valve prolapse, and dilated cardiomyopathy. Two types of accessory pathways (AP) exist: In *manifest* AP, antegrade conduction occurs over the AP and results in pre-excitation on baseline ECG (which may be intermittent). In *concealed* AP, antegrade conduction occurs via the AV node, and retrograde conduction occurs over the AP; thus pre-excitation is not evident on the baseline ECG. Approximately 50% of patients with WPW manifest tachyarrhythmias, of which 80% is AV reentry tachycardia, 15% is atrial fibrillation, and 5% is atrial flutter. Asymptomatic individuals have an excellent prognosis. For patients with recurrent tachycardias, the overall prognosis is good, but in rare instances sudden death may occur. The presence of delta waves and secondary repolarization abnormalities can lead to false positive or false negative diagnoses of ventricular hypertrophy, bundle branch block, or acute myocardial infarction. The polarity of the delta waves can be used to predict the location of the bypass tract.

35. AV DISSOCIATION

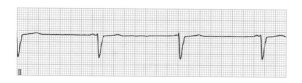

- Atrial and ventricular rhythms are independent of each other.
- Ventricular rate is usually ≥ atrial rate.

  Note: AV dissociation is a secondary phenomenon resulting from some other disturbance of cardiac rhythm.

- AV dissociation may involve:

  ‣ A ventricular rate that is faster than the normal atrial rate because of acceleration of a subsidiary pacemaker (e.g., junctional or ventricular tachycardia, myocardial ischemia, digitalis toxicity, postoperative state)

  ‣ A ventricular rate that is faster than the normal atrial rate because of slowing of the atrial rate (sinus bradycardia, sinus arrest, sinoatrial exit block, high vagal tone, post-cardioversion, β-blockers) below the intrinsic rate of a subsidiary AV junctional or ventricular pacemaker

  ‣ A ventricular rate that is slower than the atrial rate because of AV block

Abnormalities of QRS Axis

36. LEFT AXIS DEVIATION

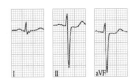

* Mean QRS axis between –30° and –90°

  Note: Causes include:
  ‣ Left anterior fascicular block (if axis > –45°, item 45)
  ‣ Inferior wall MI (items 57, 58)
  ‣ LBBB (item 47)
  ‣ LVH (item 40)
  ‣ Ostium primum ASD (item 79)
  ‣ Chronic lung disease (item 81)
  ‣ Hyperkalemia (item 74)

37. RIGHT AXIS DEVIATION

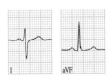

- Mean QRS axis between 100° and 270°

  Note: Causes include:

  ‣ RVH (item 41)

  ‣ Vertical heart

  ‣ Chronic lung disease (item 81)

  ‣ Pulmonary embolus (item 82)

  ‣ Left posterior fascicular block (item 46)

  ‣ Lateral wall myocardial infarction (items 55, 56)

  ‣ Dextrocardia (item 80)

  ‣ Lead reversal (item 3)

  ‣ Ostium secundum ASD (item 78)

38. ELECTRICAL ALTERNANS

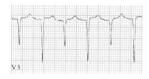

- Alternation in the amplitude and/or direction of P, QRS, and/or T waves

  Note: Causes include:

  ‣ Pericardial effusion (item 83)

  Note: Electrical alternans is due to swinging of the heart in the pericardial fluid during the cardiac cycle. Only one-third of patients with QRS alternans have a pericardial effusion, and only 12% of patients with pericardial effusions have QRS alternans. If electrical alternans involves the entire P-QRS-T ("total alternans"), effusion with tamponade is often present (which is almost always associated with sinus tachycardia).

- ‣ Severe heart failure
- ‣ Hypertension
- ‣ Coronary artery disease
- ‣ Rheumatic heart disease
- ‣ Supraventricular or ventricular tachycardia
- ‣ Deep respirations

QRS Voltage Abnormalities

39. LOW VOLTAGE

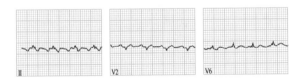

- Amplitude of the entire QRS complex (R + S) < 10 mm in all precordial leads and < 5 mm in all limb leads.

  Note: Causes include:
  - ‣ Chronic lung disease (item 81)
  - ‣ Pericardial effusion (item 83)
  - ‣ Obesity
  - ‣ Restrictive or infiltrative cardiomyopathies

- ‣ Coronary disease with extensive infarction of the left ventricle
- ‣ Myxedema (item 87)
- ‣ Pleural effusion

40. LEFT VENTRICULAR HYPERTROPHY

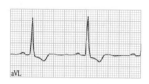

Voltage criteria for LVH (sufficient for diagnosis without repolarization abnormalities)

- **Cornell Criteria** (most accurate)—R wave in aVL + S wave in V_3:
    - ‣ > 28 mm in males
    - ‣ > 20 mm in females
- **Other commonly used voltage-based criteria**
    - ‣ **Precordial leads** (one or more of the following):
        - • R wave in V_5 or V_6 + S wave in V_1:
            - • > 35 mm if age > 40 years
            - • > 40 mm if age 30–40 years
            - • > 60 mm if age 16–30 years
        - • Maximum R wave + S wave in precordial leads > 45 mm

- R wave in $V_5 > 26$ mm
- R wave in $V_6 > 20$ mm
› **Limb leads** (one or more of the following):
  - R wave in lead I + S wave in lead II ≥ 26 mm
  - R wave in lead I ≥ 14 mm
  - S wave in aVR ≥ 15 mm
  - R wave in aVL ≥ 12 mm (a highly specific finding, except when associated with left anterior fascicular block)
  - R wave in aVF ≥ 21 mm

Note: The amplitude of the QRS (and sensitivity for the diagnosis of LVH by voltage criteria) is often decreased by conditions that increase the amount of body tissue (obesity), air (COPD, pneumothorax), fluid (pericardial or plural effusion), or fibrous tissue (coronary artery disease, sarcoid or amyloid of the heart) between the myocardium and ECG electrodes. Severe RVH can also underestimate the ECG diagnosis of LVH by canceling prominent QRS forces from the thickened LV. Left bundle branch block may also reduce QRS amplitude as well. In contrast, thin body habitus, left mastectomy, LBBB, WPW, and left anterior fascicular block may increase QRS amplitude in the absence of LVH, decreasing the specificity of the voltage criteria.

Nonvoltage-related changes (often present but not required for the diagnosis of LVH)

- Left atrial abnormality/enlargement (item 6)
- Left axis deviation (item 36)

- Nonspecific intraventricular conduction disturbance (item 49)
- Delayed onset of intrinsicoid deflection (beginning of QRS to peak of R wave > 0.05 second)
- Small or absent R waves in V_1–V_3 (low anterior forces)
- Absent Q waves in leads I, V_5, V_6
- Abnormal Q waves in leads II, III, aVF (due to left axis deviation)
- Prominent U waves (item 69)
- R wave in V_6 > V_5, provided there are dominant R waves in these leads

Repolarization (ST and/or T wave) abnormalities suggesting LVH (see item 67)

41. RIGHT VENTRICULAR HYPERTROPHY

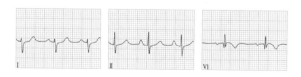

- Right axis deviation with mean QRS axis $\geq +100°$
- Dominant R wave
  - R/S ratio in V_1 or V_3R > 1, *or* R/S ratio in V_5 or V_6 $\leq$ 1
  - R wave in V_1 $\geq$ 7 mm
  - R wave in V_1 + S wave in V_5 or V_6 > 10.5 mm
  - rSR′ in V_1 with R′ > 10 mm
  - qR complex in V_1

- Secondary ST-T changes (downsloping ST depression, T-wave inversion) in right precordial leads (if present, be sure to code) (item 67)

- Right atrial abnormality/enlargement (item 5) common

- Onset of intrinsicoid deflection (beginning of QRS to peak of R wave) in V_1 < 0.05 second

   Note: For ECG features of RVH in the setting of chronic lung disease, see item 81.

   Note: Severe RVH can also underestimate the ECG diagnosis of LVH by canceling prominent QRS forces from the thickened LV.

   Note: Conditions that can present with right axis deviation and/or a dominant R wave and possibly mimic RVH include:

   ‣ Posterior or inferoposterolateral wall MI (items 59, 60). When a tall R wave is present in lead V_1, other ECG findings can help distinguish right ventricular hypertrophy (RVH) from posterior MI: T-wave inversions in V_1 and V_2 and right axis deviation favor the diagnosis of RVH, while inferior Q waves suggestive of inferior MI favor the diagnosis of posterior MI.

   ‣ Right bundle branch block (items 43, 44)

   ‣ Wolff-Parkinson-White syndrome (type A) (item 34)

   ‣ Dextrocardia (item 80)

   ‣ Left posterior fascicular block (item 46)

   ‣ Normal variant (especially in children)

42. COMBINED VENTRICULAR HYPERTROPHY

Suggested by any of the following:

- ECG meets one or more diagnostic criteria for LVH (item 40) and RVH (item 41)
- Precordial leads show LVH but QRS axis is > 90°
- LVH plus:
  - ‣ R wave > Q wave in aVR, *and*
  - ‣ S wave > R wave in V_5, *and*
  - ‣ T-wave inversion in V_1
- Large-amplitude, equiphasic (R=S) complexes in V_3 and V_4 (Katz-Wachtel phenomenon)
- Right atrial abnormality/enlargement (item 5) with LVH pattern (item 40) in precordial leads

Intraventricular Conduction Abnormalities

43. RBBB, COMPLETE

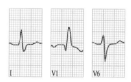

I   V1   V6

- Prolonged QRS duration (≥ 0.12 second)
- Secondary R wave (R′) in leads V_1 and V_2 (rsR′ or rSR′) with R′ usually taller than the initial R wave

- Delayed onset of intrinsicoid deflection (beginning of QRS to peak of R wave > 0.05 second) in V_1 and V_2

- Secondary ST and T-wave changes (T-wave inversion; downsloping ST segment may or may not be present) in leads V_1 and V_2

- Wide, slurred S wave in leads I, V_5, and V_6

   Note: In RBBB, mean QRS axis is determined by the initial unblocked 0.06–0.08 second of QRS and should be normal unless left anterior fascicular block (item 45) or left posterior fascicular block (item 46) is present.

   Note: RBBB does not interfere with the ECG diagnosis of left ventricular hypertrophy or Q-wave MI.

   Note: Can be seen in:

   ‣ Occasionally in normal adults (incidence ~ 2/1000) without underlying structural heart disease (unlike LBBB). These patients have essentially the same prognosis as the general population. However, among patients with coronary artery disease, RBBB is associated with a twofold increase in morality (compared to patients with coronary disease but without bundle branch block).

   ‣ Hypertensive heart disease

   ‣ Myocarditis

   ‣ Cardiomyopathy

   ‣ Rheumatic heart disease

   ‣ Cor pulmonale (acute or chronic)

‣ Degenerative disease of the conduction system (Lenègre disease) or sclerosis of the cardiac skeleton (Lev disease)

‣ Ebstein anomaly

44. RBBB, INCOMPLETE

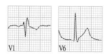

• RBBB morphology (rSR′ in V_1, item 43) with a QRS duration between 0.09 and 0.12 second

Note: Other causes of RSR′ pattern < 0.12 second in lead V_1 include:

‣ Normal variant (present in ~ 2% of healthy adults) (item 2)

‣ Right ventricular hypertrophy (item 41)

‣ Posterior wall MI (items 59, 60)

‣ Incorrect lead placement (electrode for lead V_1 placed in 3rd instead of 4th intercostal space) (item 3)

‣ Skeletal deformities (e.g., pectus excavatum)

‣ Atrial septal defect (items 78, 79)

45. LEFT ANTERIOR FASCICULAR BLOCK

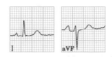

- Left axis deviation with mean QRS axis between $-45°$ and $-90°$ (item 36)
- qR complex (or an R wave) in leads I and aVL
- rS complex in lead III
- Normal or slightly prolonged QRS duration (0.08–0.10 second)
- No other factors responsible for left axis deviation:
  ‣ LVH (item 40)
  ‣ Inferior wall MI (items 57, 58)
  ‣ Emphysema (chronic lung disease) (item 81)
  ‣ Left bundle branch block (item 47)
  ‣ Ostium primum atrial septal defect (item 79)
  ‣ Severe hyperkalemia (item 74)

Note: LAFB may result in a false-positive diagnosis of LVH based on voltage criteria in leads I or aVL.

Note: Poor R-wave progression is common.

Note: Left anterior fascicular block can mask the presence of inferior wall MI.

Note: When QS complexes are present in the inferior leads, inferior MI and LAFB may both be present, but inferior MI alone should be coded.

Note: The anterior fascicle of the left bundle branch supplies the Purkinje fibers to the anterior and lateral walls of the left ventricle.

Note: Seen in organic heart disease, congenital heart disease, and rarely in normals.

46. LEFT POSTERIOR FASCICULAR BLOCK

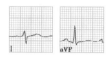

- Right axis deviation with mean QRS axis between +100° and +180° (item 37)
- Normal or slightly prolonged QRS duration (0.08–0.10 second)
- No other factors responsible for right axis deviation:
    ‣ RVH (item 41)
    ‣ Vertical heart
    ‣ Emphysema (chronic lung disease) (item 81)
    ‣ Pulmonary embolus (item 82)
    ‣ Lateral wall MI (items 55, 56)
    ‣ Dextrocardia (item 80)
    ‣ Lead reversal (item 3)
    ‣ Wolff-Parkinson-White pattern (item 34)

Note: Left posterior fascicular block can mask the presence of lateral wall MI.

Note: Compared to the left anterior fascicle, the left posterior fascicle is shorter, thicker, and receives blood supply from both left and right coronary arteries. Isolated left posterior fascicular block (LPFB) is much less prevalent than left bundle branch block, right bundle branch block, or left anterior fascicular block.

Note: Coronary artery disease is the most common cause of LPFB; when it develops during acute MI, multivessel coronary disease and extensive infarction are usually present, and the prognosis is poor. LPFB is rarely seen in normals.

47. LBBB, COMPLETE

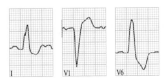

- Prolonged QRS duration (≥ 0.12 second)
- Delayed onset of intrinsicoid deflection (i.e., beginning of QRS to peak of R wave > 0.05 second) in leads I, V_5, V_6
- Broad monophasic R waves in leads I, V_5, V_6 that are usually notched or slurred
- Secondary ST and T-wave changes opposite in direction to the major QRS deflection (i.e., ST depression and T-wave inversion in leads I, V_5, V_6; ST elevation and upright T wave in leads V_1 and V_2)
- rS or QS complex in right precordial leads

Note: Left axis deviation may be present (item 36).

Note: LBBB interferes with determination of QRS axis and identification of ventricular hypertrophy and acute MI. Although the formal diagnosis of LVH should not be made in the setting of LBBB, echocardiographic and pathological studies show that ~ 80% of patients with LBBB have abnormally increased LV mass.

Note: Seen in:

▸ LVH (item 40)

▸ Myocardial infarction

▸ Organic heart disease

▸ Congenital heart disease

▸ Degenerative conduction system disease

▸ Rarely in normals

48. LBBB, INCOMPLETE

- LBBB morphology (item 47) with a QRS duration ≥ 0.09 second and < 0.12 second

49. NONSPECIFIC INTRAVENTRICULAR CONDUCTION DISTURBANCE

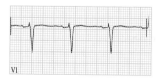

- QRS ≥ 0.11 second in duration but morphology does not meet criteria for LBBB (item 47) or RBBB (item 43), *or*

- Abnormal notching of the QRS complex without prolongation

  Note: Nonspecific IVCD may be seen with:
  ‣ Antiarrhythmic drug toxicity (especially type IA and IC agents) (item 73)
  ‣ Hyperkalemia (item 74)
  ‣ LVH (item 40)
  ‣ Wolff-Parkinson-White pattern (item 34)
  ‣ Hypothermia (item 88)
  ‣ Severe metabolic disturbances

50. FUNCTIONAL (RATE-RELATED) ABERRANT INTRAVENTRICULAR CONDUCTION

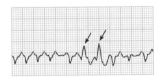

- Wide (> 0.12 second) QRS complex rhythm due to under-lying supraventricular arrhythmia, such as atrial fibrillation, atrial flutter, other SVTs

  Note: Since the right bundle has a longer refractory period than the left bundle, aberrant conduction usually occurs down the left bundle, resulting in QRS morphology with RBBB pattern.

  Note: May resemble VT (see item 25 for criteria to distinguish between SVT with aberrancy and VT).

Note: Return to normal intraventricular conduction may be accompanied by T-wave abnormalities.

Q-Wave Myocardial Infarctions

Myocardial Ischemia vs. Injury vs. Infarction

- Ischemia: ST-segment depression; T waves usually inverted; Q waves absent
- Injury: ST-segment elevation; Q waves absent
- Infarction: Abnormal Q waves; ST-segment elevation or depression; T waves inverted, normal, or upright and symmetrically peaked

  Note: Prior MI may be present without Q waves in:

  1. Anterior MI: May only see low anterior R-wave forces with decreasing R-wave progression in leads V_2–V_5.
  2. Posterior MI: Dominant R wave in V_1 and/or V_2, usually in the setting of inferior MI. ST depression is often present during acute infarction in leads V_1–V_3.

Significant ST Elevation

- New ST-segment elevation at the J point (where QRS complex meets the ST segment) in ≥ 2 contiguous leads

  ST elevation ≥ 2 mm in leads V_1, V_2, or V_3

  ST elevation ≥ 1 mm in other leads
- Usually with upwardly convex ("out-pouching") configuration
- Can persist 48 hours to 4 weeks after MI

Note: Persistent ST elevation beyond 4 weeks suggests the presence of a ventricular aneurysm.

T-Wave Inversion

Typically begins while the ST segments are still elevated (in contrast to pericarditis) and may persist indefinitely.

Note: Acute infarction can occur without significant ST-segment elevation or depression; up to 40% of patients with acute occlusion of the left circumflex coronary artery and 10–15% of patients with right coronary artery or left anterior descending artery occlusions may not have significant ECG changes.

Abnormal Q Waves

- Any Q wave in leads V_2–V_3
- Q wave ≥ 0.03 second in leads I, II, aVL, aVF, V_4, V_5, or V_6
- Q-wave changes must be present in at least two contiguous leads and must be ≥ 1 mm in depth.

    Note: The presence of a Q wave cannot be used to reliably distinguish transmural from subendocardial MI.

    Note: Abnormal Q waves regress or disappear over months to years in up to 20% of patients with Q-wave MI.

Age of Infarct Can Be Approximated from the ECG

- *Age recent or acute*: The repolarization abnormalities associated with acute myocardial infarction typically evolve in a relatively predictable fashion. Usually, the earliest finding is marked peaking of the T waves (*hyper-acute T waves*) in the region of the infarct; these are often missed since they occur very early (< 15 minutes) in the course of the acute event and are transient. If transmural ischemia persists for more than a few minutes, the peaked T waves evolve into *ST-segment elevation*, which should be ≥ 1 mm in height to be considered significant. The ST-segment elevation of myocardial infarction is usually upwardly **convex** (in contrast to acute pericarditis or normal variant early repolarization, in which the ST elevation is usually upwardly **concave**). As the acute infarction continues to evolve, the ST-segment elevation decreases and the *T waves begin to invert*. The T waves usually become progressively deeper as the ST-segment elevation subsides. *Abnormal Q waves* develop within the first few hours to days after an infarction.

› Acute MI: Abnormal Q waves, ST elevation (associated ST depression is sometimes present in noninfarct leads). Hyperacute (tall, peaked) T waves are seen very early (transient).

› Recent MI: Abnormal Q waves, isoelectric ST segments, ischemic (usually inverted) T waves are present.

• *Age indeterminate or old*: Abnormal Q waves, isoelectric ST segments, nonspecific or normal T waves

Note: Exception: MI may be present without Q waves in:

1. Anterior MI: May only see low anterior R-wave forces with decreasing R-wave progression in leads V_2–V_5.

2. Posterior MI: Dominant R wave and ST depression in leads V_1–V_3.

Pseudoinfarction Pattern

See pages 43–44 for conditions causing pseudoinfarcts (ECG pattern mimicking myocardial infarction).

Diagnosis of Q-Wave MI in the Presence of Bundle Branch Block

- RBBB: Does not interfere with the diagnosis of Q-wave MI; Q-wave criteria apply for all infarctions.
- LBBB: Difficult to diagnose any infarct in the presence of LBBB. However, acute injury is sometimes apparent.

51. ANTEROLATERAL MI (AGE RECENT OR ACUTE)

- Abnormal Q waves with significant ST-segment elevation in leads V_4–V_6

52. ANTEROLATERAL MI (AGE INDETERMINATE OR OLD)

- Abnormal Q waves in leads V_4–V_6 *without* significant ST-segment elevation

53. ANTERIOR OR ANTEROSEPTAL MI (AGE RECENT OR ACUTE)

- Abnormal Q waves with significant ST-segment elevation in at least two consecutive leads between V_2 and V_4

  Note: The presence of a Q wave in V_1 distinguishes anteroseptal from anterior infarction, although the distinction between the two is not necessary for testing purposes.

Note: Many ECG texts consider decreasing R-wave voltage from V_2 to V_5 consistent with age indeterminate anterior MI, even in the absence of abnormal Q waves. However, because the board score sheet lists the various MIs under the subheading of "Q-wave infarction," loss of R-wave voltage in the precordial leads in the absence of abnormal Q waves should not be coded as an MI.

54. ANTERIOR OR ANTEROSEPTAL MI (AGE INDETERMINATE OR OLD)

- Abnormal Q waves in at least two consecutive leads between V_2 and V_4 *without* significant ST-segment elevation

55. LATERAL MI (AGE RECENT OR ACUTE)

- Abnormal Q waves with significant ST-segment elevation in leads I and aVL

   Note: An isolated Q wave in aVL does not qualify as a lateral MI.

56. LATERAL MI (AGE INDETERMINATE OR OLD)

- Abnormal Q waves in leads I and aVL *without* significant ST-segment elevation

57. INFERIOR MI (AGE RECENT OR ACUTE)

- Abnormal Q waves with significant ST-segment elevation in at least two of leads II, III, aVF

   Note: Associated ST depression is usually evident in leads I, aVL, V_1–V_3.

58. INFERIOR MI (AGE INDETERMINATE OR OLD)

* Abnormal Q waves in at least two of leads II, III, aVF *without* significant ST-segment elevation

59. POSTERIOR MI (AGE RECENT OR ACUTE)

* Initial R wave ≥ 0.04 second in V_1 or V_2 with R-wave amplitude $\geq$ S-wave amplitude (R/S > 1) and significant (usually ≥ 2 mm) ST-segment depression
  ‣ Upright T waves are usually evident in same leads as dominant R wave.

Note: The posterior wall of the left ventricular differs from the anterior, inferior, and lateral walls by not having ECG leads directly overlying it. Instead of Q waves and ST elevation, acute posterior MI presents with mirror-image changes in the anterior precordial leads (V_1–V_3), including dominant R waves (the mirror-image of abnormal Q waves), and horizontal ST-segment depression (the mirror-image of ST elevation). Acute posterior infarction is often associated with ECG changes of acute inferior or inferolateral myocardial infarction, but may occur in isolation.

Note: RVH (item 41), WPW (item 34), and RBBB (item 43) may interfere with the ECG diagnosis of posterior MI.

60. POSTERIOR MI (AGE INDETERMINATE OR OLD)

- Dominant R wave (R/S > 1) in leads V_1 or V_2 without significant ST-segment depression

  Note: Must be distinguished from other causes of a tall R wave in leads V_1 or V_2, including RVH, WPW, RBBB, and incorrect electrode placement.

  Note: Evidence of inferior wall ischemia or infarction is often present.

Repolarization Abnormalities

61. NORMAL VARIANT, EARLY REPOLARIZATION

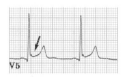

- Elevated take-off of ST segment at the junction between the QRS and ST segment (J junction)
- Concave upward ST elevation ending with a symmetrical upright T wave (often of large amplitude)

  Note: ST elevation should be less than 25% of the height of the T wave in lead V_6.

- Distinct notch or slur on downstroke of R wave
- Most commonly involves V_2–V_5; sometimes II, III, aVF

- No reciprocal ST-segment depression

  Note: Some degree of ST elevation is present in the majority of young healthy individuals, especially in the precordial leads.

62. NORMAL VARIANT, JUVENILE T WAVES

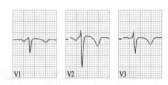

- Persistently negative T waves (usually not symmetrical or deep) in leads V_1–V_3 in normal adults
- T waves still upright I, II, V_5, V_6

  Note: Juvenile T waves is a normal variant ECG finding commonly seen in children, occasionally seen as a normal variant in adult women, but only rarely seen in adult men.

63. NONSPECIFIC ST AND/OR T-WAVE ABNORMALITIES

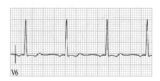

- Slight (< 1 mm) ST depression or elevation, *and/or*
- T wave that is flat or slightly inverted

  Note: Normal T waves usually ≥ 10% the height of R wave

  Note: Can be seen in:

  › Organic heart disease

  › Drugs (e.g., quinidine)

  › Electrolyte disorders (e.g., hyperkalemia, hypokalemia)

  › Hyperventilation

  › Myxedema (item 87)

  › Recent large meal

  › Stress

  › Pancreatitis

  › Pericarditis (item 84)

  › CNS disorders (item 86)

  › LVH (item 40)

  › RVH (item 41)

  › Bundle branch block (items 43, 47)

  › Healthy adults (normal variant) (item 2)

  › Persistent juvenile pattern: T-wave inversion in V_1–V_3 in young adults

64. ST AND/OR T-WAVE ABNORMALITIES SUGGESTING MYOCARDIAL ISCHEMIA

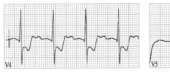 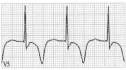

- Ischemic ST-segment changes:
  - ‣ Horizontal or downsloping ST segments with or without T-wave inversion

  Note: Flutter waves or prominent atrial repolarization waves (as can be seen in left/right atrial enlargement, pericarditis, atrial infarction) can deform the ST segment and result in pseudodepression.

- Ischemic T-wave changes:
  - ‣ Biphasic T waves with or without ST depression
  - ‣ Symmetrical or deeply inverted T waves; QT interval often prolonged

  Note: Reciprocal T-wave changes may be evident (e.g., tall, upright T waves in inferior leads with deeply inverted T waves in anterior leads).

  Note: T waves may become less inverted or upright during acute ischemia (pseudonormalization).

  Note: Prominent U waves (upright or inverted) (item 69) are often present.

  Note: Tall upright T waves may also be seen in:
  - ‣ Normal healthy adults (item 2)
  - ‣ Hyperkalemia (item 74)

- ‣ Early myocardial infarction
- ‣ LVH (item 40)
- ‣ CNS disorders (item 86)
- ‣ Anemia

65. ST AND/OR T-WAVE ABNORMALITIES SUGGESTING MYOCARDIAL INJURY

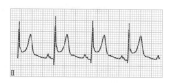

- Acute ST-segment elevation ≥ 1 mm with upward convexity (may be concave early) in the leads representing the area of jeopardized myocardium/acute infarction.

- ST and T-wave changes evolve: T waves invert before ST segments return to baseline.

- Associated ST depression in the noninfarct leads is common.

- Acute posterior wall injury often has horizontal or downsloping ST-segment depression with upright T waves in V_1 and/or V_2 with prominent R wave in these same leads.

    Note: It is important to consider the clinical context, since ST-segment elevation suggesting myocardial injury can also be seen in:

    - ‣ Acute pericarditis (item 84)
    - ‣ Ventricular aneurysm

- Early repolarization (item 61)
- LVH (item 40)
- Hyperkalemia (item 74)
- Bundle branch block (items 43, 47)
- Myocarditis
- Apical hypertrophic cardiomyopathy (item 85)
- Central nervous system disorder (item 86)
- Normals (ST elevation up to 3 mm may be seen in leads V_1–V_3)

66. ST AND/OR T-WAVE ABNORMALITIES SUGGESTING ELECTROLYTE DISTURBANCES

- Any abnormalities suggesting hyperkalemia, hypokalemia, hypercalcemia, or hypocalcemia (see items 74–77)

  Note: Hypomagnesemia causes changes similar to hypocalcemia (QT prolongation).

  Note: Renal failure often results in multiple electrolyte derangements with a wide variety of associated ECG abnormalities.

67. ST AND/OR T-WAVE ABNORMALITIES SECONDARY TO HYPERTROPHY

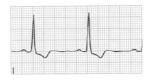

- **LVH**: ST segment and T-wave displacement opposite to the major QRS deflection:
  - ST depression (upwardly concave) and T-wave inversion when the QRS is mainly positive (leads I, V_5, V_6)
  - Subtle (< 1 mm) ST elevation and upright T waves when the QRS is mainly negative (leads V_1, V_2); with more extreme voltage, ST elevation up to 2–3 mm can be seen in leads V_1–V_2
- **RVH**: ST-segment depression and T-wave inversion in leads V_1–V_3 and sometimes in leads II, III, aVF

68. PROLONGED QT INTERVAL

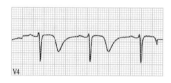

- Corrected QT interval (QTc) ≥ 0.45 second in males and females, where *QTc = QT when the heart rate is 60 bpm = QT interval divided by the square root of the preceding R-R interval*

  Note: Be sure to measure the QT interval in a lead with a large T wave and distinct termination. Also look for the lead with the longest QT.

- Easier method to determine QT interval:
  - Use 0.40 second as the normal QT interval for a heart rate of 70. For every 10 bpm change in heart rate above (or below) 70, subtract (or add) 0.02 second.

(Measured value should be within ± 0.04 second of the calculated normal.) *Example:* For a heart rate of 100 bpm, the calculated normal QT interval = 0.40 second – (3 × 0.02 second) = 0.34 ± 0.04 second. For a heart rate of 50 bpm, the calculated normal QT interval = 0.40 second + (2 × 0.02 second) = 0.44 ± 0.04 second.

‣ In general, the normal QT interval should be less than 50% of the R-R interval.

Note: The QT interval represents the period of ventricular electrical systole (i.e., the time required for ventricular depolarization and repolarization to occur), varies inversely with heart rate, and is longer while asleep than while awake (presumably due to vagal hypertonia).

Note: Conditions associated with a prolonged QT interval include:

‣ Drugs (quinidine, procainamide, disopyramide, amiodarone, sotalol, dofetilide, azimilide, phenothiazines, tricyclics, lithium)

‣ Hypomagnesemia

‣ Hypocalcemia (item 77)

‣ Marked bradyarrhythmias

‣ Intracranial hemorrhage (item 86)

‣ Myocarditis

‣ Mitral valve prolapse

‣ Myxedema (item 87)

‣ Hypothermia (item 88)

- ‣ Very high-protein diets
- ‣ Romano-Ward syndrome (congenital; normal hearing)
- ‣ Jervell and Lange-Nielsen syndrome (congenital; deafness)

69. PROMINENT U WAVES

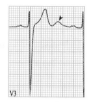

- Amplitude ≥ 1.5 mm

  Note: The U wave is normally 5–25% the height of the T wave and is largest in leads V_2 and V_3.

  Note: Causes include:

  - ‣ Hypokalemia (item 75)
  - ‣ Bradyarrhythmias
  - ‣ Hypothermia (item 88)
  - ‣ LVH (item 40)
  - ‣ Coronary artery disease
  - ‣ Drugs (digitalis, quinidine, amiodarone, isoproterenol)

Suggested Clinical Disorders

70. DIGITALIS EFFECT

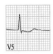

- Sagging ST-segment depression with upward concavity
- T wave flat, inverted, or biphasic
- QT interval shortened
- U-wave amplitude increased
- PR interval lengthened

Note: ST changes are difficult to interpret in the setting of LVH, RVH, or bundle branch block. However, if typical sagging ST segments are present and the QT interval is shortened, consider digitalis effect.

71. DIGITALIS TOXICITY

- Digitalis toxicity can cause almost any type of cardiac dysrhythmia or conduction disturbance except bundle branch block. Typical abnormalities include:
  - ▸ Paroxysmal atrial tachycardia with block
  - ▸ Atrial fibrillation with complete heart block (regular R-R intervals)
  - ▸ Second- or third-degree AV block

‣ Complete heart block (item 33) with accelerated junctional rhythm (item 22) or accelerated idioventricular rhythm (item 26)

‣ Supraventricular tachycardia with alternating bundle branch block

Note: Digitalis toxicity may be exacerbated by hypokalemia, hypomagnesemia, and hypercalcemia.

Note: Electrical cardioversion of atrial fibrillation is contraindicated in the setting of digitalis toxicity since protracted asystole or ventricular fibrillation can occur. (Digitalis levels should always be checked prior to elective electrical cardioversion.)

72. ANTIARRHYTHMIC DRUG EFFECT

Suggested by the following:

- Mild prolongation of QT interval (item 68)
- Prominent U waves (one of the earliest findings) (item 69)
- Nonspecific ST and/or T-wave abnormalities (item 63)
- Decrease in atrial flutter rate

73. ANTIARRHYTHMIC DRUG TOXICITY

Suggested by the following:

- Marked prolongation of QT interval (item 68)
- Ventricular arrhythmias including torsade de pointes (paroxysms of irregular ventricular tachyarrhythmia at a rate of 200–280 bpm with sinusoidal cycles of changing QRS amplitude and polarity in the setting of a prolonged QT interval)

- Wide QRS complex
- Various degrees of AV block
- Marked sinus bradycardia (item 9), sinus arrest (item 11), or sinoatrial exit block (item 12)

74. HYPERKALEMIA

ECG changes depend on serum K^+ level and rapidity of rise:

- **K^+ = 5.5–6.5 mEq/L**
  - ‣ Tall, peaked, narrow-based T waves

    Note: Generally defined as > 10 mm in precordial leads and > 6 mm in limb leads; may also be seen as normal variant or in acute MI, LVH, or LBBB
  - ‣ QT interval shortening
  - ‣ Reversible left anterior fascicular block (item 45) or left posterior fascicular block (item 46)
- **K^+ = 6.5–7.5 mEq/L**
  - ‣ First-degree AV block (item 29)
  - ‣ Flattening and widening of the P wave
  - ‣ QRS widening
- **K^+ > 7.5 mEq/L**
  - ‣ Disappearance of P waves, which may be caused by:
    - Sinus arrest (item 11), *or*
    - Sinoventricular conduction (sinus impulses conducted to the ventricles via specialized atrial fibers *without* atrial depolarization)
  - ‣ LBBB (items 47, 48), RBBB (items 43, 44), or markedly widened and diffuse intraventricular con-

duction disturbance (item 49) resembling a sine-wave pattern

‣ ST-segment elevation

‣ Arrhythmias and conduction disturbances including ventricular tachycardia (item 25), ventricular fibrillation (item 28), idioventricular rhythm (items 26, 27), asystole

75. HYPOKALEMIA

Suggested by the following:

• Prominent U waves (item 69)

• ST-segment depression and flattened T waves

   Note: The ST-T and U-wave changes of hypokalemia are seen in approximately 80% of patients with potassium levels < 2.7 mEq/L, compared to 35% of patients with levels of 2.7–3.0 mEq/L, and 10% of patients with levels > 3.0 mEq/L.

• Increased amplitude and duration of the P wave

• Prolonged QT sometimes seen

   Note: If potassium replacement does not normalize the QT interval, suspect hypomagnesemia.

• Arrhythmias and conduction disturbances, including paroxysmal atrial tachycardia with block, first-degree AV block (item 29), type I second-degree AV block (item 30), AV dissociation (item 35), VPCs (item 23), ventricular tachycardia (item 25), and ventricular fibrillation (item 28)

76. HYPERCALCEMIA

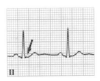

- QTc shortening (usually due to shortening of the ST segment)
- May see PR prolongation

  Note: Little if any effect on P, QRS, or T wave.

77. HYPOCALCEMIA

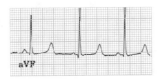

- Prolonged QTc (item 68) (earliest and most common finding) due to ST-segment prolongation without changing the duration of the T wave (seen only with hypocalcemia or hypothermia)
- Occasional flattening, peaking, or inversion of T waves

78. ATRIAL SEPTAL DEFECT, SECUNDUM

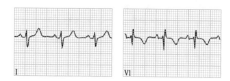

Suggested by the following:

- Typical RSR′ or rSR′ complex in V$_1$ with a QRS duration < 0.11 second (incomplete RBBB, item 44)
- Right axis deviation (item 37) ± right ventricular hypertrophy (item 41)
- Right atrial abnormality/enlargement (item 5) in ~ 30%
- First-degree AV block (item 29) in < 20%

    Note: Ostium secundum ASDs represent 70–80% of all ASDs; they are due to deficient tissue in the region of the fossa ovalis.

79. ATRIAL SEPTAL DEFECT, PRIMUM

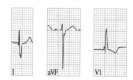

Suggested by the following:

- RSR′ complex in V$_1$
- Incomplete RBBB (item 44)

- Left axis deviation (item 36) (in contrast to right axis deviation in ostium secundum ASD)
- First-degree AV block (item 29) in 15–40%
- Advanced cases have combined ventricular hypertrophy (item 42).

Note: Ostium primum ASDs represent 15–20% of all ASDs and are due to deficient tissue in the lower portion of the septum. These ASDs are usually large and may be accompanied by anomalous pulmonary venous drainage. Primum ASDs are often associated with a cleft anterior mitral valve leaflet, mitral regurgitation, and Down syndrome.

80. DEXTROCARDIA, MIRROR IMAGE

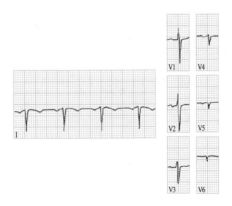

Suggested by the following:

- P-QRS-T in leads I and aVL are inverted ("upside-down")

  Note: Dextrocardia and lead reversal (item 3) can both produce an upside-down P-QRS-T in leads I and aVL. To distinguish between these conditions, look at the R-wave pattern in V_1–V_6:

  ‣ Reverse R-wave progression (i.e., decreasing R-wave amplitude from leads V_1–V_6) suggests dextrocardia.

  ‣ Normal R-wave progression suggests lead reversal.

  Note: In ***mirror-image dextrocardia***, the most common form of dextrocardia, the abdominal and thoracic viscera (in addition to the heart) are transposed to the side opposite their usual locations (dextrocardia with "situs inversus"). This form of dextrocardia is generally not associated with severe congenital cardiac abnormalities (other than the malposition, which does not affect cardiac function). In ***isolated dextrocardia***, the heart is rotated to the right side of the chest, but other viscera remain in their usual locations. This type of dextrocardia is almost always associated with serious congenital cardiac abnormalities, resulting in clinical difficulties in infancy or early childhood.

81. CHRONIC LUNG DISEASE

- ECG features suggestive of COPD include:
  ‣ Right ventricular hypertrophy (item 41)
  ‣ Right axis deviation (item 37)
  ‣ Right atrial abnormality/enlargement (item 5)
  ‣ Poor precordial R-wave progression

- Low voltage (item 39)
- Pseudo-anteroseptal infarct pattern (low anterior forces)
- S waves in leads I, II, and III (S1S2S3 pattern)
- May also see sinus tachycardia (item 10), junctional rhythm (item 22), multifocal atrial tachycardia (item 16), various degrees of AV block, nonspecific IVCD (item 49), or bundle branch block (items 43, 44, 47, 48)

  Note: Right ventricular hypertrophy in the setting of chronic lung disease is suggested by:
  - Rightward shift of QRS
  - T-wave inversion in V_1, V_2
  - ST depression in leads II, III, aVF
  - Transient RBBB
  - RSR′ or QR complex in V_1

82. ACUTE COR PULMONALE INCLUDING PULMONARY EMBOLUS

- ECG changes often accompany large pulmonary emboli and are associated with elevated pulmonary artery pressures, right ventricular dilation and strain, and clockwise rotation of the heart:
  - S_1Q_3 or $S_1Q_3T_3$ occurs in up to 30% of cases and lasts for 1–2 weeks.
  - Right bundle branch block (incomplete or complete) may be seen in up to 25% of cases and usually lasts less than 1 week.

‣ Inverted T waves secondary to right ventricular strain may be seen in the right precordial leads and can last for months.

‣ Other ECG findings include right axis deviation, non-specific ST and T-wave changes, and P pulmonale.

‣ Arrhythmias and conduction disturbances include sinus tachycardia (most common arrhythmia), atrial fibrillation, atrial flutter, atrial tachycardia, and first-degree AV block.

• The clinical presentation and ECG of acute pulmonary embolus may sometimes be confused with acute inferior MI: Q waves and T-wave inversions may be seen in leads III and aVF in both conditions; however, a Q wave in lead II is uncommon in pulmonary embolus and suggests MI.

Note: ECG abnormalities are often *transient*, and a normal ECG may be recorded despite persistence of the embolus. Sinus tachycardia, however, is usually present even when other ECG features of acute cor pulmonale are absent.

83. PERICARDIAL EFFUSION

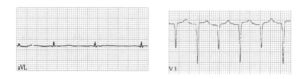

• Low-voltage QRS (item 39) (left strip) and/or electrical alternans (item 38) (right strip)

Note: Low-voltage QRS complexes and electrical alternans are consistent with (but not very sensitive or specific for) the diagnosis of pericardial effusion.

- Other features of acute pericarditis (item 84) may or may not be present.

84. ACUTE PERICARDITIS

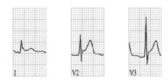

- Classic evolutionary ST and T-wave pattern consists of four stages (but is not always present):
  - ▸ Stage 1: Upwardly concave ST-segment elevation in almost all leads except aVR; no reciprocal ST depression in other leads except aVR.
  - ▸ Stage 2: ST junction (J point) returns to baseline, and T-wave amplitude begins to decrease.
  - ▸ Stage 3: T waves invert.
  - ▸ Stage 4: ECG returns to normal.

Note: T-wave inversion usually occurs *after* the ST segment returns to baseline (in contrast to myocardial infarction, where T-wave inversion typically begins while the ST segments are still elevated).

Note: Pericarditis may be focal (e.g., postpericardiotomy) and result in regional (rather than diffuse) ST elevation.

Note: Classic ST and T-wave changes are more likely to occur in purulent pericarditis as opposed to idiopathic, rheumatic, or malignant pericarditis.

- Other clues to acute pericarditis include:
  - ‣ Sinus tachycardia (item 10)
  - ‣ PR depression early (PR elevation in aVR)
  - ‣ Low voltage (item 39)
  - ‣ Electrical alternans (item 38) if pericardial effusion (item 83)

85. HYPERTROPHIC CARDIOMYOPATHY

- Majority have abnormal QRS
  - ‣ Large-amplitude QRS
  - ‣ Large abnormal Q waves (can give pseudoinfarct pattern in inferior, lateral, and anterior precordial leads)
  - ‣ Tall R wave with inverted T wave in V_1 simulating RVH
- Left axis deviation (item 36) in 20%
- ST and T-wave changes
  - ‣ Nonspecific ST and/or T-wave abnormalities are common (item 63)
  - ‣ ST and/or T-wave changes secondary to ventricular hypertrophy or conduction abnormalities
  - ‣ Apical variant of hypertrophic cardiomyopathy has deep T-wave inversions in V_4–V_6 (item 85)
- Left atrial abnormality/enlargement (item 6) is common; right atrial abnormality/enlargement (item 5) on occasion

Note: The vast majority of patients with hypertrophic cardiomyopathy have abnormal ECGs, with LVH in 50–65%, left atrial abnormality/enlargement in 20–40%, and pathological Q waves (especially leads I, aVL, V_4–V_5) in 20–30%. ST and T-wave changes (repolarization abnormalities secondary to LVH) are the most common ECG findings, while right axis deviation is rare. Sinus node disease and AV block are occasional manifestations of this disorder. The most frequent cause of mortality is sudden death, with risk factors including young age and a history of syncope and/or asymptomatic ventricular tachycardia on ambulatory monitoring.

86. CENTRAL NERVOUS SYSTEM DISORDER

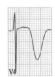

- "Classic changes" of cerebral and subarachnoid hemorrhage usually occur in the precordial leads:
    ‣ Large upright or deeply inverted T waves
    ‣ Prolonged QT interval (often marked) (item 68)
    ‣ Prominent U waves (item 69)
- Other changes:
    ‣ T-wave notching with loss of amplitude
    ‣ ST-segment changes:

- Diffuse ST elevation mimicking acute pericarditis, *or*
- Focal ST elevation mimicking acute myocardial injury, *or*
- ST depression
  ‣ Abnormal Q waves mimicking MI
  ‣ Almost any rhythm abnormality (sinus tachycardia or bradycardia, junctional rhythm, VPCs, ventricular tachycardia, etc.)

Note: ECG findings in CNS disease can mimic those of:
  ‣ Acute myocardial infarction
  ‣ Acute pericarditis (item 84)
  ‣ Drug effect or toxicity (items 70–73)

87. MYXEDEMA

- Low voltage (item 39)
- Sinus bradycardia (item 9)
- T wave flattened or inverted
- PR interval may be prolonged (item 29)
- Frequently associated with pericardial effusion (item 83)
- Electrical alternans (item 38) possible

88. HYPOTHERMIA

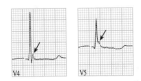

- Sinus bradycardia (item 9)
- Prolongation of PR, QRS, and QT (items 29, 49, 68)
- Osborne ("J") wave: Late upright terminal deflection of QRS complex ("camel hump" sign); amplitude increases as temperature declines

  Note: Notching simulating an Osborne wave may be seen in early repolarization

- Atrial fibrillation (item 19) in 50–60%
- Other arrhythmias include AV junctional rhythm (item 22), ventricular tachycardia (item 25), ventricular fibrillation (item 28)

89. SICK SINUS SYNDROME

One or more of the following:

- Marked sinus bradycardia (item 9)
- Sinus arrest (item 11) or sinoatrial exit block (item 12)
- Bradycardia alternating with tachycardia
- Atrial fibrillation with slow ventricular response preceded or followed by sinus bradycardia, sinus arrest, or sinoatrial exit block

- Prolonged sinus node recovery time after atrial premature complex or atrial tachyarrhythmias
- AV junctional escape rhythm
- Additional conduction system disease is often present, including AV block (items 29–33), nonspecific IVCD (item 49), and/or bundle branch block (items 43, 44, 47, 48).

Paced Rhythms

90. ATRIAL OR CORONARY SINUS PACING

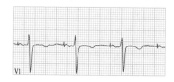

- Pacemaker stimulus followed by an atrial depolarization
- If the rate of the intrinsic rhythm falls below that of the pacemaker, atrial-paced beats occur and will be separated by a constant (A-A) interval.
- Appropriately sensed intrinsic atrial activity (P wave) resets pacemaker timing clock. After an interval of time (A-A interval) with no sensed atrial activity, an atrial-paced beat occurs.

91. VENTRICULAR DEMAND PACEMAKER (VVI), NORMALLY FUNCTIONING

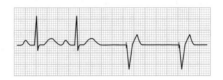

- Pacemaker stimulus followed by a QRS complex of different morphology than intrinsic QRS
- A ventricular demand (VVI) pacemaker senses and paces only in the ventricle and is oblivious to native atrial activity. If constant ventricular pacing is noted throughout the tracing, it is impossible to distinguish ventricular demand from asynchronous ventricular pacing. Thus, the diagnosis of ventricular demand pacing requires evidence of appropriate inhibition of pacemaker output in response to a native QRS (at least one).
- Appropriately sensed ventricular activity (QRS complex) resets pacemaker timing clock. After an interval of time (V-V interval) with no sensed ventricular activity, a ventricular-paced beat is delivered and a new cycle begins.
- A spontaneous QRS arising before the end of the V-V interval is sensed and the ventricular output of the pacemaker is inhibited. A new timing cycle begins.
- For rate-responsive VVI-R pacemakers, ventricular-paced rate increases with activity (up to a defined upper rate limit).

92. DUAL-CHAMBER PACEMAKER (DDD)

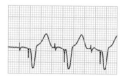

- Atrial and ventricular pacing and sensing
- *For atrial sensing*, need to demonstrate inhibition of atrial output and/or triggering of ventricular stimulus in response to intrinsic atrial depolarization
- If pacemaker rate exceeds rate of intrinsic rhythm, there will be atrial (A)- and ventricular (V)-paced beats with defined intervals between the A and V spikes (A-V interval) and from the V spike to the subsequent A spike (V-A interval).
- Following V-sensed activity (either QRS or paced [V] beats), the timing clock is reset. If intrinsic atrial activity (P) is sensed prior to the end of the V-A interval, atrial output of the pacemaker will be inhibited. If no intrinsic atrial activity (P) is sensed by the end of the V-A interval, an atrial-paced beat will occur.

Following atrial-sensed activity (either intrinsic [P] or paced [A] beats), the timing clock is reset. If intrinsic ventricular activity (QRS) is sensed prior to the end of the AV interval, ventricular output of the pacemaker will be inhibited. If no intrinsic ventricular activity (QRS) is sensed by the end of the A-V interval, a ventricular-paced beat will occur.

93. PACEMAKER MALFUNCTION, NOT CONSTANTLY CAPTURING (ATRIUM OR VENTRICLE)

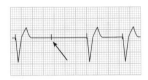

- Pacing spike is not followed by appropriate depolarization (at a time when myocardium is not refractory).
- May be due to lead displacement, perforation, increased pacing threshold (from MI, flecainide, amiodarone, hyperkalemia), lead fracture or insulation break, pulse generator failure (from battery depletion), or inappropriate reprogramming.

  Note: Rule out "pseudomalfunction" (i.e., pacer stimulus falls into refractory period of ventricle).

94. PACEMAKER MALFUNCTION, NOT CONSTANTLY SENSING (ATRIUM OR VENTRICLE)

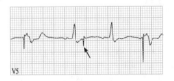

- Pacemaker in "inhibited" mode: Failure of pacemaker to be inhibited by an appropriate intrinsic depolarization
- Pacemaker in "triggered" mode: Failure of pacemaker to be triggered by an appropriate intrinsic depolarization
- Pacemaker timing is not reset by intrinsic or ectopic beat, resulting in asynchronous firing of pacemaker (paced rhythm competes with the intrinsic rhythm)
- Occurs with low-amplitude signals (especially VPCs) and inappropriate programming of the sensitivity. All causes of failure to capture (item 93) can also cause failure to sense.

Note: Can often be corrected by reprogramming the sensitivity of the pacemaker.

Note: Watch for "pseudomalfunction" (i.e., pacer stimulus falls into refractory period of ventricle).

Note: Premature depolarizations may not be sensed if they:

- ▸ Fall within the programmed refractory period of the pacemaker
- ▸ Have insufficient amplitude at the sensing electrode site

Note: Any stimulus falling early within the QRS complex probably does not represent sensing malfunction; commonly seen with right ventricular electrodes in RBBB.

INDEX

ECGs and figures are indicted by page numbers in italics. Tables are indicated by t following the page number.

Index

Index

Index

Index

Index

Index

Index